Obsessive Compulsive Disorder

Obsessive Compulsive Disorder

Stuart Montgomery
*St Mary's Hospital Medical School,
London, UK*

Joseph Zohar
*Chaim Sheba Medical Center and
Sackler School of Medicine,
Tel Aviv University Israel,
Tel Hashomer*

MARTIN DUNITZ

First published in the United Kingdom in 1999 by
Martin Dunitz Ltd
The Livery House
7– 9 Pratt Street
London NW1 0AE

A CIP record for this book is available from the British Library.

ISBN 1-85317-387-8

Printed and bound by The Friary Press
Dorchester, Dorset

Contents

What is obsessive compulsive disorder?

Obsessive compulsive disorder (OCD) is a distinctive and frequently disabling illness characterized by unwanted thoughts that recur (obsessional ruminations) and unwanted repetitive acts that the patient realizes are foolish but is unable to resist (compulsive rituals). The thoughts and behaviours are not a source of pleasure although they may serve to reduce discomfort. This is not the 'obsessional' or 'compulsive' of common parlance used to describe, for example, the meticulous, or the house-proud. The obsessions or compulsions, which may be resisted at least initially, cause marked distress, are time-consuming, and interfere with social functioning, when severe sufferers may be preoccupied with the obsessional behaviours for much of the day and unable to pursue their normal activities.

Although systematic clinical investigation of OCD began relatively recently, the condition has been recognized for centuries and descriptions of what would be regarded as classical OCD occur as early as the sixteenth century. In the seventeenth century the distressing, unwanted thoughts Bishop John Moore describes are like those that trouble OCD sufferers:

'[they have] naughty, and sometimes Blasphemous Thoughts [which] start in their Minds, while they are exercised in the Worship of God [despite] all their endeavours to stifle and suppress them the more they struggle with them, the more they increase'.

Lady Macbeth in Shakespeare's play exemplifies compulsive washing, one of the most common compulsive behaviours in OCD:

'it is an accustomed action with her, to seem thus washing her hands. I have known her continue with this a quarter of an hour' (Macbeth, V.i.28).

Until relatively recently OCD was thought to be a rare condition affecting some 0.05% of the population. However, the considerable research interest that has been focused on the condition in the last ten to fifteen years has shown it to be much more common than was previously thought. As a result of large epidemiological studies it is now known that OCD is among the most frequently occurring psychiatric disorders affecting more than 50 million persons worldwide. OCD is a serious illness with high costs to both the individual and society and the higher than hitherto recognized prevalence, therefore, has important consequences.

The burden of the illness

OCD is a disorder with an early age of onset, often in early childhood. Very few studies have been carried out with repeated measures over years to establish the course of the illness and it is therefore not well understood how many sufferers may recover, or to what extent they improve. It is, however, clear that in a substantial proportion of cases OCD runs a chronic, fluctuating course with exacerbations. It thus represents a total sum of suffering of immense proportion to the individuals, both from the disorder and from the limitations it imposes on their daily lives.

Many of those with OCD also have symptoms of other psychiatric disorders. Depressive symptoms are frequent and two thirds of those with OCD have depressive symptoms that would fulfil criteria for major depression. OCD can be life threatening and there is an increased suicide attempt rate compared with the normal population. The rate is even higher in those with OCD and a comorbid psychiatric diagnosis, even when major depression, which itself carries an increased suicide risk, is excluded (Hollander et al 1997).

OCD can have a devastating effect on the family, who are often drawn in to 'assisting' with the obsessional behaviours. As a result the activities of the family become as constrained as those of the member with OCD. The sufferer's relationships, both within the family and with friends and colleagues, are often very adversely affected.

The distress to the individual and those near to him or her and the costs to the sufferer and to society arising from the disorder were brought into vivid focus in a survey of some 700 OCD sufferers carried out recently in the USA. OCD was seen to have a major impact on many areas of life. The disorder was reported to have affected the education of sufferers, their ability in the workplace, and their relationships. The majority has lowered their career aspirations and many were unable to work at all because of their OCD symptoms. The economic implications for sufferers and their families as well as for society are serious (Table 1).

Activity	% reporting interference
Decrease in self-esteem	92.1
Lowered career aspirations	66.3
Negative relationship with spouse	64.4
Fewer friends	62.1
Decrease in academic achievement	60.1
Negative effect on relationship with parent	59.8
Involvement of family member in symptoms	57.8
Thinking about suicide	57.1
Negative effect on relationship with child	51.7
Change of career or job	47.7
Loss of an intimate relationship	42.9
Interfered with social function of family member	33.1
Interfered with job of family member	26.1
Led to break-up of marriage/relationship	23.7
Laid off from work	22.4
Led to alcohol abuse	18.6
Led to abuse of other drugs	13.1
Suicide attempt	12.2
Interfered with academic performance of family member	9.3

Adapted from Hollander et al 1997

Table 1
Interference in social function due to OCD reported in a survey of 700 sufferers in the USA.

OCD sufferers are often very isolated; they fear to speak of their problems with anybody lest others consider them to be mad. It is a common phenomenon for OCD patients to have suffered for more than ten years before presenting for professional assistance. In view of the far-reaching consequences of

OCD for the individual, this reluctance to call for help is perhaps surprising. However, many are unaware that their condition is amenable to medical treatment.

The considerable progress that has been made in the last fifteen years in identifying specific antiobsessional drugs, in developing new effective treatments for OCD, and in refining psychological treatment programmes has advanced the understanding of the disorder and improved the hopes of a better quality of life for sufferers.

Epidemiology of OCD

Prevalence

Until 1984, the most widely quoted figure regarding the prevalence of OCD symptoms in the general population was 0.05%. However, the early studies were not carried out on a representative sample, being based on the relatively small number of patients who were so severely ill that hospitalization was the only alternative. These studies underestimated the prevalence of OCD in the community, which, though it did not reach medical attention, or if it did, was not deemed appropriate for hospitalization, was severe enough to cause substantial impairment. More recent studies have been carried out on large samples in the general population and a very much higher prevalence is generally reported. The seminal Epidemiological Catchment Area Study carried out in a sample of 18 000 in the community found a prevalence of approximately 2% (Robins et al 1984, Karno et al 1988) (Table 2).

A large crossnational epidemiological study by Weissmann et al in 1994, which examined the prevalence of OCD, was unique in using similar methods and diagnostic criteria in seven different countries (the USA, Canada, Puerto Rico, Germany, Taiwan, Korea, and New Zealand) and over four continents (ie

Disorder	Prevalence rate over lifetime (%)
Major depressive disorder	5.2
Obsessive compulsive disorder	2.5
Schizophrenia	1.6
Panic disorder	1.4
Severe cognitive impairment	1.2
Anorexia nervosa	0.1
From Robins et al 1984	

Table 2
Prevalence of psychiatric disorder in USA Epidemiological Catchment Area Survey.

America, Europe, Asia, and Australia). The prevalence of OCD was found to be approximately 2% in the USA, Canada, and Puerto Rico and the rates observed in Europe, New Zealand, and Asia were remarkably consistent. Only in one site, Taiwan, was the prevalence of OCD lower, at 0.7%, parallelling the low incidence of all psychiatric disorders in Taiwan (Figure 1; Table 3). These findings establish OCD as a common disorder with a prevalence placed between that of major depressive disorder and schizophrenia.

Is there some geographic variation in the prevalence of OCD? Although the very low rate reported in Taiwan (0.7%) may be explained by the overall low rate of reported psychiatric disorder, another study carried out in India has also reported a similar low rate (0.6%). Sociodemographic factors on the other hand appear to have little influence on the prevalence of OCD and studies that have investigated this possibility have found no correlation with race, socioeconomic status, or educational

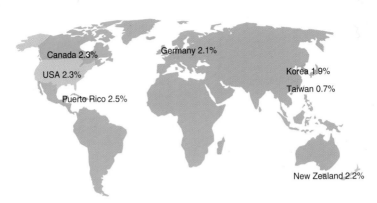

Figure 1
Prevalence of OCD worldwide. (Adapted from Weissman et al 1994.)

Study	Location	Prevalence (%)
Robins et al 1984	USA	2.5
Bland et al 1988	Canada	3.0
Karno et al 1988	USA	2.5
Zohar et al 1992a	Israel	3.6*
Reinherz et al 1993	USA	2.1*
Chen et al 1993	Hong Kong	2.1
Lindal and Stefannson 1993	Iceland	2.0
Weissman et al 1994	USA	2.3
	Canada	2.3
	Puerto Rico	2.5
	Germany	2.1
	Taiwan	0.7
	Korea	1.9
	New Zealand	2.2
Valleni-Basile et al 1994	USA	3.0

From Weissman et al 1994
* Adolescent sample

Table 3
Prevalence of OCD worldwide.

level either in adolescents or adults (Flament et al 1988, Karno and Golding 1991).

If the prevalence of OCD worldwide is of the order of 2% the total number of patients who suffer from the disorder can be estimated as at least 50 million, which defines OCD as a global problem.

The reported prevalence rates are likely to be affected by the diagnostic instrument used and by the threshold level set to identify cases. It has become apparent from the epidemiological studies which have used internationally accepted diagnostic criteria with clear definitions to identify cases that there is a sizeable group who do not meet full diagnostic criteria for OCD but have a subclinical disorder. This group is described in longitudinal studies in adults and may be as large as the group with the full disorder (Degonda et al 1993). In the study of adolescents in the USA of Valeni-Basile et al (1994) the prevalence of those with subclinical disorder was 19%. This may be an important group in whom the subclinical condition may develop into full OCD, since a study in adults shows that an individual may vary above and below the threshold for OCD at different times (Degonda et al 1993).

Age of onset

OCD has an early age of onset with a mean age of between 19 and 20 years. Retrospective studies have found that between 30% and 50% of adults report that their symptoms started in childhood or adolescence. The figure may well be higher given the unreliability of retrospective memory. Specific studies of the incidence of OCD in young people have identified lifetime prevalence rates similar to those reported in adult population samples. For example a rate of 2% was reported in a study of high-school students in the USA (Flament et al 1988) and a higher rate of 3.6% in a group of 16–17-year-old army recruits in Israel (Zohar et al 1992a). A similar rate (3%) was reported in a recent study of a community sample of more than 3000 adolescents who were followed up over a two-year period in the USA (Valleni-Basile et al 1994).

Cultural aspects

The prevalence of OCD appears to be remarkably constant across geographical and cultural boundaries but the question arises whether cultural factors influence the presentation of the disorder. Transcultural comparisons between Europe and the USA have found few crosscultural differences that mostly related to the *content* of the obsession, while the phenomenology remains the same across locations as varied as the USA, India, England, Japan, Denmark, and Israel. The most common obsession in these six countries, regardless of specific cultural background, appears to be the obsession about dirt or contamination. The second most common obsession is fear of producing harm or aggression, the third is somatic, the fourth, religious, and the fifth, sexual obsessions.

	USA (*n*=425)	India (*n*=410)
Dirt/ contamination	38	32
Harm/ aggression	24	20
Somatic	7	24
Religious	6	5
Sexual	6	6

Table 4
Content of obsessions in different countries (%).

The cultural influence on the *content* of the obsessions has been noted in the epidemiological studies. A study carried out in Egypt of OCD symptomatology in sufferers of different religious belief including Christians, Hindus, Muslims, and Jews found, as other epidemiological studies have done, that the commonest obsession related to contamination in all groups but that the contamination was related to varying religious themes (Okasha et al 1994). There is some risk that OCD may be missed if certain behaviours, which are in fact manifestations of OCD, are considered as being appropriate within a religious context.

It seems that while cultural, religious, and historical background can influence the specific content of obsessions, the core themes and compulsions remain the same. For example, throughout the present century, patients with OCD have been obsessed at different times with the plague, leprosy, tuberculosis, syphilis, and, most recently, AIDS. Yet the core ritual or compulsion — washing — endured (Table 4).

UK (*n*=86)	Japan (*n*=61)	Denmark (*n*=61)	Israel (*n*=34)
47	39	34	50
47	12	23	20
	13	18	3
5		8	9
10	5	6	6

Clinical picture of OCD

Symptom clusters of OCD

The symptoms of OCD, which at a cursory glance might appear to be of great diversity, fall into a limited number of broad categories. The most frequently occurring obsessions relate, as has already been mentioned, to a fear of contamination, then doubt, need for symmetry, aggressive and sexual thoughts. The most frequently occurring compulsions are checking, then washing, counting, rituals related to the need for symmetry and hoarding (Table 5).

Fear of contamination

The most prevalent obsession is concerned with contamination by dirt and/or germs. Typically, patients with this obsessional symptom cluster attempt to avoid sources of 'contamination' such as door-knobs, electric switches, newspapers, dirt on the street, etc. Washing is the accompanying compulsion and such patients may spend several hours daily washing their hands, showering, or cleaning. Paradoxically, some of these patients

Obsessions	%	Compulsions	%
Contamination	45	Checking	60
Pathological doubt	42	Washing	50
Somatic	36	Counting	36
Need for symmetry	31	Need to ask or confess	31
Aggressive impulse	28	Symmetry/precision	28
Sexual impulse	26	Hoarding	18
Other	13	Multiple compulsions	48
Multiple obsessions	60		

From Rasmussen and Tsuang 1986

Table 5
Symptoms of 250 OCD patients admitted for treatment.

are actually quite slovenly. They may refuse to touch even their own bodies, knowing that if they do, they will not be at ease unless they carry out extensive washing rituals.

An example of a public figure who displayed OCD symptoms of a fear of dirt is the legendary Howard Hughes. Hughes sought to avoid any contact with insects to the extent that dinner parties and business meetings would be halted whilst insects that might have crept in were found and destroyed. He was obsessed with avoiding germs. He feared contamination and avoided touching anyone or anything. When contact could not be avoided he devised a system of 'insulations' of paper towels and tissues for protection and even telephone conversations were conducted through a protective paper barrier placed over the mouthpiece. To protect against germs he demanded that everything be brought to him wrapped in special tissues. He also insisted that doors and windows be sealed in order to prevent germs from entering his home. He took ever-increasing precautions against germs in his houses, and crockery used by guests had to be destroyed after their departure. Ultimately, Hughes was overwhelmed by these efforts and ended his life in filth and neglect (Figure 2).

- Was obsessed with avoiding germs since childhood
- Devised 'insulations' of paper towels and tissues for protection, and demanded that anything brought to him was wrapped in special tissue
- Insisted that doors and windows be sealed
- Was ultimately overwhelmed by his efforts and ended his life in filth and neglect

---

Figure 2
Businessman Howard Hughes.

Checking

The second major symptom cluster is checking. These patients are obsessed with doubt, usually tinged with guilt, and are frequently concerned that if they do not check carefully enough they will harm others. Yet instead of resolving uncertainty, their repeated checking often only contributes to even greater doubt, which leads to further checking. Often these patients will enlist the help of family and friends to ensure they have checked enough or correctly. By some inscrutable means, the checker ultimately resolves a particular doubt, only to have it replaced by a new one. Resistance, which in this case involves the attempt to refrain from checking, leads to difficulty in concentrating and to exhaustion from the endless intrusion of nagging uncertainties.

Common examples of such doubts are the fear of leaving the door unlocked that leads to checking it over and over, fear of causing a fire that leads to checking the stove (even to the extent that the patient cannot leave home, or the fear of hurting someone while driving, leading to repetitive driving back over the same spot after hitting a bump in the road. Some checkers may not even be sure why they are checking; they feel they are merely led by the inexplicable 'urge' to do so.

Checkers may also engage in related compulsive behaviours. Sometimes, uncertain whether the checking is sufficient, patients may develop 'undoing' or protective rituals such as counting to a certain number in their head, repeating actions a specific number of times, or avoiding particular numbers.

Pure obsessions

The obsessional patient with pure obsessions experiences repetitive, intrusive thoughts, which are usually somatic, aggressive, or sexual, and are always reprehensible to the thinker. Sexual obsessions include forbidden or perverse sexual thought, images, or impulses that may involve children, animals, incest, homosexuality, etc.

Discrete and obvious compulsive ritualistic behaviours may be absent but these obsessions might be considered as 'mental compulsions'. The obsessions are often associated with fearful images or thoughts of aggressive or sexual impulses directed at a person valued by the patient. There may be a fear of acting on other impulses (for example killing someone, robbing a bank, or stealing) or a fear of being held responsible for some terrible event (for example fire, plague, war).

Subtle rituals often accompany these obsessive thoughts. For example a mother who is afraid she will stab her daughter may struggle with this impulse by avoiding knives, then sharp objects, and ultimately by avoiding touching her daughter.

Although such avoidant behaviour may not be perceived immediately as an actual repetitive behaviour or compulsion, it shares other properties of compulsion in that it is carried out in an intentional attempt to 'neutralize' the obsession.

Obsessional thoughts may also be of a religious rather than sexual or violent nature. Such thoughts can lead to repetitive silent prayer or confession or result in more apparent rituals such as repeated bowing or trips to temple, church, or synagogue. This behaviour presents a particular problem to clinicians and to clergy as they attempt to draw the line between disorder and devotion.

Order and symmetry

Checking behaviour is also a frequent component of a different type of obsessive compulsive symptom, a concern with order, symmetry, and touching. Patients feel profoundly uncomfortable if they are unable to follow a particular sequence of actions related to ordinary daily activities, or if particular objects are misplaced. They are driven to check that everything is correctly positioned before they can function, however time-consuming and impeding the checking may be. Or they may feel driven to touch certain things however inappropriate the action.

Charles Dickens is recorded in a recent biography as having to walk right around his house and grounds checking that everything was in its rightful place, including pictures and books, before being able to start a day's work. Certain objects, including a particular paper knife and small statue, had to be on his desk before he could start writing and work would be delayed if they were not available. He also had a touching compulsion and would comb his hair even at socially inappropriate moments, going through the performance 'a hundred times a day' as a colleague in late life reported.

Contemporary reports about the eighteenth-century literary figure, Dr Samuel Johnson, show him to have suffered from obsessional symptoms involved with touching. Johnson's biographer reports that he made 'extraordinary gestures or antics with his hands when passing over the threshold of a door', that he refused to step on cracks between paving stones, and that he touched every post he passed on a walk, going back if he happened to miss one. For Johnson, such symptoms led to a great deal of suffering and, despite the recognition of his genius, Boswell, Johnson's biographer, notes that these and other unusual habits led to a certain isolation from society.

Obsessional slowness

Obsessional slowness manifests itself in patients with the obsession when they have to have objects or events in a certain order or position, to do and undo certain motor actions in an exact way, or to have things perfectly symmetrical or 'just right'. Such patients require an inordinate amount of time to complete even the simplest of tasks: thus merely getting dressed may take a couple of hours. Unlike most obsessive-compulsive patients, these patients usually do not resist their symptoms. Instead, they seem to be consumed with completing their routine precisely. Although this subtype of OCD is relatively rare, aspects of slowness often appear along with other obsessions and compulsions and may be the major source of interference in daily functioning.

Hoarding

A less frequent, but disabling OCD symptom is hoarding. Patients with hoarding as the predominant obsessional symptom pattern appear to make little attempt to resist their symptoms. They may refuse to throw out anything — junk mail, old newspapers, used tissues, broken furniture, food past its sell by date — because they fear throwing away something important in the process.

Not being able to bear to throw anything away may afflict many people in its milder forms. For example the actor Lord Laurence Olivier has been reported to have held on compulsively to everything — used tickets, recipes, licences, and, most of all, letters. However, in OCD the behaviour comes to interfere with daily living. Sufferers have complete indecision as to whether something is finished with; they fear to throw anything away in case they might need it later and often suffer acute distress for considerable periods if they do manage to throw something out. The result is that old items and possessions begin to accumulate until the person's home is completely filled. Some individuals even move to bigger homes and proceed to fill those too. Simple activities like getting dressed become difficult because clothes are piled too high to reach a particular garment. Domestic tasks like preparing food take inordinate amounts of effort and time because reaching the kitchen becomes an exhausting obstacle course. Patients are often embarrassed and shamed by their behaviour, which they find to be a huge burden.

Combinations of symptoms

Many OCD patients have a combination of symptoms, although one symptom type, be it washing, checking pure obsessions, or obsessional slowness, may predominate. Patients report that different OCD symptoms are predominant at different points in the course of their illness. Thus a patient who in childhood may have had predominantly washing rituals may have checking rituals as an adult. The principal reason for noting this symptom shift is not in terms of treatment but in order to increase the level of confidence in making the OCD diagnosis.

OCD is associated with significant pain and distress. Patients are well aware that their obsessions and compulsions do not make sense, and most attempt to resist them at some point during the course of their illness. However, the urge to carry them out is most often overwhelming. This discrepancy between the knowledge that such obsessions and compulsions are irrational and the overpowering urge to perform them contributes to the immense suffering associated with the disorder.

Diagnosing OCD

Identifying the patient with OCD

The symptoms of OCD are very clear and easily identified. If OCD is indeed so prevalent a psychiatric disorder, why then do we still not diagnose OCD more often? Part of the answer to this question lies in the ego-dystonic nature of the disorder. Patients will often attempt to disguise their symptoms due to the shame or embarrassment associated with the disorder. Thus, they will not reveal their obsessive-compulsive symptoms unless asked about them directly.

In order to identify an OCD sufferer, therefore, every mental status examination should include five specific questions about OCD (see Table 6). Unless these five questions are asked the diagnosis of OCD patients is likely to elude the clinician since, unless they are directly questioned, these patients are unlikely to reveal their symptoms.

Diagnosing the OCD is of crucial importance because specific antiobsessional treatments are now available (to be discussed later) and many patients will show substantial improvement in their obsessive-compulsive symptoms and in their quality of life (Koran et al 1996), and will experience a significant decrease in suffering.

1 Do you wash or clean a lot?
2 Do you check things a lot?
3 Is there any thought that keeps bothering you that you would like to get rid of but can't?
4 Do your daily activities take a very long time to finish?
5 Are you concerned about orderliness or symmetry?

Table 6
Five questions to help identify an OCD sufferer.

Diagnostic criteria

Diagnostic criteria for OCD on Axis I of DSM-IV (Diagnostic and Statistical Manual — American Psychiatric Association 1995) include the presence of recurrent, persistent, and unwanted thoughts, impulses, or images (obsessions) and/or the performance of repetitive, often seemingly purposeful, ritualistic behaviours (compulsions). The ego-dystonic nature of the illness, the attempt to resist, and interference with daily function are also mandatory for diagnosis (Table 7).

Diagnostic issues

There is some divergence between the two main accepted diagnostic classifications as to the nature of OCD. The DSM-IV classifies OCD as part of the anxiety disorders which include phobias (specific and social), panic disorder (with and without agoraphobia), post-traumatic stress disorder, generalized anxiety disorder due to a medical condition or substance abuse, and acute stress disorders. In the European tradition OCD has always been considered as a separate nosological entity.

A Either obsessions or compulsions

Obsessions as defined by (1), (2), (3), and (4):

1 recurrent and persistent thoughts, impulses, or images that are experienced, at some time during the disturbance, as intrusive and inappropriate and that cause marked anxiety or distress

2 the thoughts, impulses, or images are not simply excessive worries about real-life problems

3 the person attempts to ignore or suppress such thoughts, impulses, or images, or to neutralize them with some other thought or action

4 the person recognizes that the obsessional thoughts, impulses, or images are a product of his or her own mind (not imposed from without as in thought insertion)

Compulsions as defined by (1) and (2):

1 repetitive behaviours (eg hand washing, ordering, checking) or mental acts (eg praying, counting, repeating words silently) that the person feels driven to perform in response to an obsession, or according to rules that must be applied rigidly

2 the behaviours or mental acts are aimed at preventing or reducing distress or preventing some dreaded event or situation; however, these behaviours or mental acts either are not connected in a realistic way with what they are designed to neutralize or prevent or are clearly excessive

B At some point during the course of the disorder, the person has recognized that the obsessions or compulsions are excessive or unreasonable. **Note:** This does not apply to children

C The obsessions or compulsions cause marked distress, are time consuming (take more than 1 hour a day), or significantly interfere with the person's normal routine, occupational (or academic) functioning, or usual social activities or relationships

D If another Axis I disorder is present, the content of the sessions or compulsions is not restricted to it (eg preoccupation with food in the presence of an eating disorder; hair pulling in the presence of trichotillomania; concern with appearance in the presence of body substance use disorder; preoccupation with having a serious illness in the presence of hypochondriasis; preoccupation with sexual urges or fantasies in the presence of a paraphilia; or guilty ruminations in the presence of major depressive disorder)

Table 7
DSM IV diagnostic criteria for OCD.

E The disturbance is not due to the direct physiological effects of a substance (eg a drug of abuse, a medication) or a general medical condition

Specify if:

With poor insight: if, for most of the time during the current episode, the person does not recognize that the obsessions and compulsions are excessive or unreasonable

Source: American Psychiatric Asssociation 1994

Many OCD sufferers have marked symptoms of anxiety, both psychic and somatic, and some 60% may suffer from panic attacks (Rasmussen and Eisen, 1988). However, these symptoms are not invariably associated with the disorder and their presence is not of itself sufficient reason for categorizing OCD as an anxiety disorder. These anxiety symptoms are considered to be secondary to or part of the OCD. This approach is reflected in the ICD (International Classification of Diseases) 10 classification where OCD is considered to be a 'standing-alone' disorder, not part of the anxiety disorders.

The perception of OCD as an anxiety disorder inherent in the DSM categorization does not appear to have been based on empirical evidence, and the definition of obsessions as repetitive intrusive thoughts which *cause* marked anxiety or distress and compulsions as repetitive ritualistic behaviour *aimed* to prevent or reduce anxiety seems to put the explanation ahead of the observation. Most OCD patients report an overwhelming need to obsess or ritualize and that they suffer distress when prevented. An increase or decrease specifically in anxiety is not clearly articulated.

There are, indeed, some important differences between OCD and other anxiety disorders. These include age of onset (younger in OCD patients than in those with panic disorder), lack of response to anxiogenic and anxiolytic compounds in OCD, and selective responsivity to serotonergic medications. The long-term course of illness and the female/male ratio also differ.

Differential diagnosis

Although symptoms that appear to be obsessional and compulsive are found in a variety of psychiatric disorders, and indeed also in normal mental life, two principal features distinguish OCD. First, the symptoms are ego-dystonic — they give no pleasure — and the individual, recognizing these preoccupations to be excessive or unreasonable, attempts to ignore or suppress them. This lack of pleasure in the behaviour is an important distinction that separates OCD, the disorder, from other behaviours, which are sometimes described as compulsions such as pathological gambling, overeating, alcohol, or drug abuse and hypersexuality. These behaviours can be distinguished from compulsions, as to some degree they are experienced as pleasurable, while compulsions are not. The second differentiation is that the obsessions and the compulsions cause marked distress, are time-consuming (should occupy more than one hour per day, according to the DSM-IV), and lead to significant interference in functioning.

Phobia

The association (comorbidity) between OCD and social phobia is very high. Moreover certain patients with OCD may appear to resemble simple or social phobic individuals and may present a diagnostic problem. Patients with obsessions about contamination may even describe their problem as 'germ phobia'. Although in individual cases it may be difficult to distinguish between OCD and phobia, unlike the phobic patient, the OCD patient's fear often involves harming others rather than the self.

An individual with a fear of contamination will often develop not only washing or other contamination rituals but will also develop phobic avoidance mechanisms — not entering situations where contamination is likely. The avoidance can become extreme. Patients may seek treatment claiming they have a phobia, when in fact their avoidance is motivated by obsessions. Often, close examination of the patient history will reveal the presence of the obsession as well as other obsessive or compulsive behaviours. The phobia in these patients should be recognized as part of or secondary to the OCD. The 'phobic' element in OCD is often unavoidable. How can one avoid germs, or dirt? The 'classic' phobic objects for the phobic individual include well observed objects, such as bridges, dogs, heights, etc.

Obsessive-compulsive personality disorder

Although there may be some similarities in the diagnosis of OCD — an Axis I disorder in DSM-IV — and obsessive-compulsive personality disorder (OCPD) — an Axis II disorder — they are very far apart. Compulsive personality disorder refers to individuals afflicted with perfectionism, orderliness, and rigidity, for whom these traits are acceptable or ego-syntonic. As with OCD, issues of control play an important role in OCPD, as well as 'undoing' behaviour, intellectualization, denial, and isolation of affect.

The psychoanalytic explanation for OCD suggests that the disorder develops when these defences fail to contain the anxiety of the obsessional individual. According to this view,

OCD could be considered to be on a developmental continuum of pathology with OCPD. However, there is evidence from epidemiological studies that a substantial number of patients with OCD do not exhibit premorbid compulsive personality traits (Rasmussen and Tsuang 1984). It is now generally accepted that if an individual meets the criteria for both disorders, both diagnoses should be recorded.

Obsessions and delusions

Usually a clear distinction between psychosis and OCD can be made since, although their behaviour is based on senseless or irrational ideas, OCD sufferers generally retain full insight into the absurd nature or excessiveness of their preoccupations. Diagnosis may be difficult in very severe OCD patients who briefly relinquish the struggle against their symptoms. At such times the obsessions or compulsions may appear to shift from an unwanted and distressing intrusion to a psychotic delusion. Follow-up data suggest that such psychotic-like decompensations may occur in patients with OCD who never go on to develop schizophrenia. The term 'obsessive-compulsive psychosis' has been proposed for patients with this presentation, analogous to the association between psychotic depression and depression (Insel and Akiskal 1986). Indeed, the DSM-IV includes a subtype of OCD, 'with poor insight', which specifically refers to this status.

Comorbid depression

Many patients suffering from OCD develop comorbid psychiatric conditions. At one time in the American classification system the importance of the presence of OCD was relegated to the background if another illness was shown to have occurred before the onset of the OCD. However, DSM-IV establishes that another Axis I disorder may be present provided that the content of the obsession is unrelated to it; for example guilty thoughts in the presence of major depressive disorder would be assessed as depressive symptoms, or thoughts about food in the presence of eating disorder should not be considered symptoms of OCD. Coexisting Axis I diagnoses in primary OCD are major depressive disorder (67%), simple phobia (22%), social phobia (18%), and eating disorder (17%) (Rasmussen and Eisen 1990) (Table 8).

Diagnosis	Based on semistructured interview	Based on Schedule for Affective Disorders and Schizophrenia
Major depressive disorder	67	78
Simple phobia	22	28
Separation anxiety disorder	2	17
Social phobia	18	26
Eating disorder	17	8
Alcohol abuse (dependence)	14	16
Panic disorder	12	15
Tourette's syndrome	7	6

Based on Rasmussen and Eisen 1990

Table 8
Psychiatric disorders comorbid with OCD (lifetime, %).

It is perhaps not surprising that major depressive disorder can develop as a secondary illness in individuals who find themselves wasting long hours each day washing or checking or obsessing on a persistently recurring thought — activities which prevent them from leading fully productive lives. Depression is the most common complication of OCD. Depressive symptoms are common in OCD and as many as a third of OCD patients may fulfil the diagnostic criteria for major depression (Rasmussen and Eisen 1992). It would, however, be mistaken to give a diagnosis of depression in preference to OCD, though this undoubtedly sometimes occurs partly because of the occasional difficulty in distinguishing depressive from obsessional ruminations.

The depressive symptoms seen in OCD differ from the symptoms of major depression in a number of ways. They mirror the response of the OCD symptoms to treatment with effective antiobsessional drugs, with a relatively low rate of placebo response and slow incremental course of response. Moreover the depressive symptoms in OCD do not appear to respond to conventional antidepressants that have not shown antiobsessional efficacy. At the biological level researchers have reported some similarities in the biologic makers for depression and OCD. However, the differences between the two outweigh their similarities (see Zohar and Insel 1987 for review).

Biological substrates of OCD

From the therapeutic perspective, OCD is a unique disorder since, so far, only one type of medication — those that specifically affect the serotonergic system — appears to be beneficial. Direct comparisons of noradrenergic antidepressants with clomipramine or with selective serotonin reuptake inhibitors (SSRI) have shown the lack of antiobsessive effects of the noradrenergic drugs (Zohar et al 1992b). This selective response to medications that specifically modulate one neurotransmitter is unknown in other disorders such as depression, panic disorder, or schizophrenia. In depression and panic disorder, both noradrenergic and serotonergic reuptake blockers are effective as well as ECT (electroconvulsive therapy: for depression) and alprazolam (for panic disorder) and in schizophrenia, mixed dopaminergic and serotonergic medications seem to be effective (Table 9).

In OCD the decrease in symptomatology correlates with 5-HT indices such as changes in the metabolite of serotonin, 5-HIAA, in the cerebrospinal fluid (CSF) (Thoren et al 1980a), and reductions in serotonin activity in the platelet (Flament et al 1987) but not with the metabolite of noradrenaline, MHPG, or dopamine, HVA. Moreover, administration of a nonselective serotonin antagonist, metergoline, for four days to OCD

Study	Design	Drugs	Results
Zohar and Insel 1987	Crossover with placebo washout	DMI vs CMI	CMI>DMI DMI effect<5%
Leonard et al 1991	Crossover without placebo washout	DMI vs CMI	CMI>DMI DMI effect<10%
Goodman et al 1990	Parallel group	DMI vs FLV	FLV>DMI DMI effect<5%

Table 9
Double-blind comparisons of the noradrenergic reuptake blocker desipramine (DMI) to the serotonergic reuptake blockers clomipramine (CMI) and fluvoxamine (FLV).

patients who had responded to clomipramine reversed the antiobsessive effect (Benkelfat et al 1989). These clinical studies led to the hypothesis of OCD as a serotonergic illness.

Some additional support for the hypothesis of an abnormality of the serotonin system underlying OCD was derived from the behavioural responses observed following challenge with the serotonin agonists metachlorophenylpiperazine (mCPP), a compound with high affinity for $5\text{-}HT_{1A}$, $5\text{-}HT_{1D}$, and $5\text{-}HT_{2C}$ receptors. While the response of normal controls to oral mCPP challenge did not differ from their response to placebo, OCD patients experienced significant anxiety and depression following mCPP compared with placebo (Zohar and Insel 1987, Hollander et al 1992). A transient exacerbation of OCD symptoms was also seen in untreated patients and in some cases new or dormant symptoms emerged. The results of serotonergic challenge have not all been consistent but in general they have suggested behavioural hypersensitivity and neuroendocrine hyposensitivity to be characteristic of the OCD challenge response.

An array of 5-HT receptor subtypes has now been identified and attempts have been made to determine which subtype might be primarily implicated in OCD. So far the 5-HT_{1A} receptor appears to be ruled out by the lack of effect on OCD symptoms of the 5-HT_{1A} ligand ipsapirone (Lesch et al 1991), and also the failure of buspirone, a 5-HT_{1A} agonist, to confer added therapeutic effect when used in augmentation treatment (McDougle et al 1993). Administration of another serotonin agonist, MK-212, which has a high affinity for 5-HT_{1A} and 5-HT_{2C} receptors, also had no effects on behaviour in OCD patients (Bastani et al 1990). The 5-HT_2 receptors are involved in modulating anxiety-related behaviours and it has been suggested that the SSRIs exert an antiobsessional effect via their activity in potentiating 5-HT_2 neurotransmission — a proposal that is supported by preliminary data on the effect of clomipramine in increasing the cortisol response to 5-HTP. Moreover the antiobsessional effects of fluvoxamine are reported to be attenuated by the 5-HT_2 antagonist ritanserin. Given the findings from the mCPP, MK-212 and ipsapirone challenge studies, the 5-HT2C and 5-HT1D receptors seem more likely candidates for mediating OCD symptoms, and exacerbation of OCD symptoms with the 5-HT_{1D} agonist, sumatriptan, suggests a role for 5-HT_{1D} (Zohar 1996) (Table 10).

Although attention has been focused on the postsynaptic serotonin receptor, presynaptic mechanisms may also be implicated. The number of platelet 3H-imipramine and 3H-paroxetine binding sites, peripheral markers of the presynaptic 5-HT transporter, in drug-free OCD patients compared with

Challenge	Authors	5-HT subsystem affected	Changes in specific OC symptomatology
mCPP	Zohar et al 1987	5-HT 1A	Transient exacerbation
	Hollander et al 1992	5-HT 1D	
Ipsapirone	Lesch et al 1991	5-HT 1A	No effect
MK-212	Bastani et al 1990	5-HT 1A 5-HT 2C	No effect
Sumatriptan	Zohar 1996	5-HT 1D	Transient exacerbation

Table 10
Behavioural responses to differet serotonergic challenges.

healthy controls and patients with other anxiety disorders appears to be reduced. Treatment with an SRI brings about a significant increase in 3H-imipramine density (Marazziti et al 1992), which suggests that the 5-HT transporter may be linked to recovery and response to serotonergic drugs.

Beyond 5-HT

Although serotonin plays a major role, the pathophysiology of OCD is more complex and hence likely to involve more than a single neurotransmitter dysfunction, and other systems have come under investigation. The most compelling evidence for dopaminergic involvement in OCD comes from the clinical findings of OCD symptoms in basal ganglia disorders such as Tourette's syndrome and postencephalitic Parkinson's disease.

The close association of these disorders to OCD and the additional therapeutic benefits obtained with coadministration of dopamine blockers for one subtype of OCD — OCD with tic disorder — have suggested a role for dopaminergic dysfunction (McDougle et al 1990).

Autoimmune factors

Study of autoimmune factors has been prompted by the association of OCD and the autoimmune disease of the basal ganglia, Sydenham's chorea, a complication of rheumatic fever that is accompanied by obsessive-compulsive symptoms in over 70% of cases. In a group of children with Sydenham's chorea, 10 out of 11 had antibodies directed against human caudate tissue (Swedo et al 1993). These children had a history of OCD symptoms, which started prior to the onset of movement disorder, reached a peak in line with the motor symptoms, and declined before their resolution. Does childhood-onset OCD represent the sequelae of an antineuronal antibody-mediated response to an infectious agent such as group A haemolytic streptococcus?

A recent study following the autoimmune line of inquiry found raised serum antibodies for somatostatin and dynorphin, two of the principal neuromodulatory peptides of the basal ganglia. Much further research is needed into the possibility of an autoimmune mechanism for OCD in a subset of this population.

Brain-imaging studies

Brain-imaging research provides evidence to suggest that the underlying dysfunction in OCD is likely to be in the prefrontal cortex-basal ganglia thalamic circuitry rather than in any one single brain region. Early computerized tomography and magnetic resonance imaging studies have shown morphological changes of the basal ganglia (Luxenberg et al 1988, Scarone et al 1992). Now more sophisticated techniques such as volumetric high-resolution magnetic resonance imaging are enhancing the information available, especially with regard to the caudate nucleus.

Positron emission tomography has demonstrated abnormally high glucose metabolism in the caudate nucleus and left orbital gyri in patients with OCD compared with controls (Baxter et al 1987) and an association between OCD and increased glucose metabolism is also reported in the left orbital frontal, right sensorimotor, bilateral prefrontal, and anterior cingulate regions. This consistent orbital cortex hyperfunction in OCD differs from depression and schizophrenia, where the most replicated finding is hypofunction in the lateral prefrontal cortex.

Combining behavioural challenge with brain imaging may be a better approach to capturing brain function while the patients with OCD and control subjects are actually observed. For example, high-resolution positron emission tomography using sero-labelled CO_2 has shown that provocation of OCD symptoms in patients with OCD correlated with increasing blood flow in the left anterior orbitofrontal cortex and negatively with activation of the right posterior orbitofrontal cortex, indicating possible lateralized opposing influences of OCD symptoms (Rauch et al 1994).

Using these techniques has made it possible to identify changes in response to treatment. For example, an 18 F positron emission tomography study has shown that OCD responders showed a significant decrease in cerebral glucose metabolism in the right head of the caudate nucleus compared with pretreatment values and compared to nonresponders and normal controls in whom levels did not change (Baxter et al 1992). Similar findings have been reported in other studies. It is interesting that the effects of treatment can be measured with these methods, whether the treatment is pharmacological or behavioural.

Genetics

Since the classic report of Aubrey Lewis in 1936 several investigations have reported increased prevalence of OCD among first-degree relatives of patients with OCD. The actual rates reported have been quite variable, from 0–35%, but in general there is an increased rate suggestive of a genetic contribution. Further support for a genetic influence is provided by the greater concordance shown in monozygotic (53–87%) compared with dizygotic twins (Carey and Gottesman 1981, Rasmussen and Tsuang 1986) and from recent studies which consolidated the evidence in favour of familial involvement (Pauls et al 1995).

Summary

The serotonergic hypothesis remains a necessary but not sufficient explanation for the pathogenesis of OCD. Most evidence remains focused on the basal ganglia and on a 5-HT/dopamine inter-relationship. Given that the basal ganglia receive such rich innervation from both 5-HT and dopamine neurones, it has been postulated that OCD is subserved by a neuronal dysfunction in the basal ganglia and orbitofrontal cortex circuit. However, other systems, such as the neuropeptides arginine, vasopressin, oxytocin, and somatostatin, have also been suggested. Clinical association between obsessive-compulsive symptoms, autoimmune diseases, and D8/17 positive response in OCD patients with childhood onset of OCD, suggests the presence of an autoimmune mechanism as well. Further studies are required to understand the relevance of the serotonergic and nonserotonergic systems in different subtypes of OCD.

OCD-related disorders

A group of disorders that are characterized by obsessional thoughts or repetitive behaviours have been described as OCD spectrum disorders. The nature of the links between OCD and the individual conditions remains a source of discussion but there are certain similarities between OCD and some of the disorders included in this group.

OCD spectrum disorders, which overlap with many psychiatric diagnostic categories, include body dysmorphic disorder (BDD — dysmorphophobia), hypochondriasis, trichotillomania, eating disorders, and disorders of what is described as impulse control, covering trichotillomania, self-injurious behaviour, and sexual compulsion. A relationship is suggested with Tourette's syndrome, with autism, and with obsessional schizophrenia (McElroy et al 1994, Hollander and Wong 1995) (Figure 3). The links between this group of conditions and OCD are suggested by shared features in terms of clinical presentation, certain similarities in onset and course, similar family history of illness, or characteristic features of treatment response.

Apparent overlap with the obsessional thoughts of OCD is seen in the preoccupation with body appearance of body dysmorphic disorder, or the concern with body weight typical of

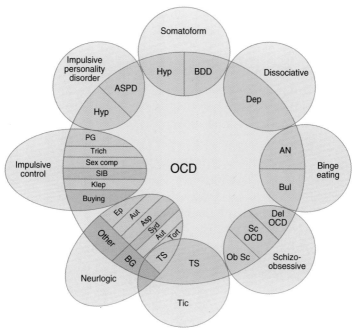

AN = anorexia nervosa
Asp = Asperger's syndrome
ASPD = antisocial personality disorder
Aut = autism
BDD = body dysmorphic disorder
BG = basal ganglia disorder
Bul = bulimia
Del OCD = delusional OCD
Dep = depersonalization disorders
Ep = epilepsy
Hyp = hypochondriasis

Klep = kleptomania
Ob Sc = obsessional schizophrenia
PG = pathological gambling
Sc OCD = schizotypical OCD
Sex comp = sexual compulsion
SIB = self-injurious behaviour
Syd = Sydenham's chorea
Tort = torticollis
Trich = trichotillomania
TS = Tourette's syndrome

Figure 3
The spectrum of OCD-related disorders. (Adapted from Hollander and Wong 1995.)

anorexia nervosa. Similarly the compulsive hair pulling of trichotillomania suggests overlap with the compulsive ritualistic behaviour of OCD. An overlap is also apparent between OCD and some of the ritualistic behaviours seen in Tourette's syndrome.

OCD is a disorder with an early onset of action, starting in many cases in early childhood, with a peak in the late teenage years or early adulthood. The OCD spectrum disorders share this early onset, appearing mainly in late adolescence. Both OCD and the OCD-related disorders tend to be long-term disorders with a chronic course. Family history also appears similar with an increased incidence of OCD and mood disorders.

Investigation of treatments of OCD-related disorders has been relatively limited. However, the results of the few studies that have been carried out indicate that some of these patients respond to the same antiobsessional agents as do OCD patients (Hollander et al 1990, Fallon et al 1993). It is possible that there may be a serotonergic component to the biological basis of these disorders.

Gilles de la Tourette's syndrome

It has been frequently observed that frank obsessional symptoms develop in a substantial proportion of patients with Gilles de la Tourette's syndrome and other movement disorders such as Sydenham's chorea (Swedo et al 1989), and a common pathway via disturbance at the basal ganglia has been postulated. The frequency of the association between OCD and Tourette's makes it unlikely to be by chance (Frankel et al 1986, Pitman et al 1987, McElroy et al 1994). A genetic component is also reported, since relatives of Tourette's patients appear to have a higher incidence of tics and OCD than the general population (17% and 12%) (Pauls et al 1986). This excess of OCD appears to be independent of whether OCD symptoms are present in the Tourette's proband or not. There is also an increased incidence of tics in OCD patients and in the families of OCD patients, suggesting a link possibly between a subgroup of OCD and Tourette's. It is, however, still unclear whether the association between OCD and Tourette's syndrome can be explained by a similar underlying pathology.

Body dysmorphic disorder (BDD)

Preoccupation with an imagined defect in one's appearance or excessive concern about a slight defect is the identifying feature of body dysmorphic disorder (BDD). The most usual complaints concern blemishes or facial flaws, the perception that a particular part of the body is abnormal in size, or that the body is asymmetrical. BDD is a fairly common condition affecting an estimated 1% of the population (Hollander and Wong 1995) though it may well be higher since it is a disorder that is largely hidden, with sufferers tending to be very secretive. Sufferers may seek medical intervention but the BDD may be missed because attention is focused on a physical problem.

Repeated reassurance that his or her appearance is normal does not satisfy the individual with BDD, and individuals frequently try to camouflage the perceived defect, often developing extensive compulsive rituals, time-consuming checking, or they may avoid social situations and become very isolated. BDD is sometimes so severe that the individual may seek surgical procedures to try to improve the troublesome perceived flaw. Individuals with BDD frequently suffer from comorbid depression and also social phobia. In patients who have been given the primary diagnosis of OCD or social phobia high levels of BDD are reported. These high rates are not seen in patients given other diagnoses of anxiety disorders such as panic disorder or generalized anxiety disorder (Brawman-Mintzer et al 1995).

Some case reports and the results of treatment studies in BDD suggest that there is a differential response to serotonergic agents as there is in OCD. Although the studies are small and lack controls to take account of possible spontaneous treatment, BDD appears to have a response to selective serotonin reuptake inhibitors but not to standard antidepressants lacking potent serotonergic action, nor to benzodiazepines or neuroleptics (Hollander 1996).

Hypochondriasis

The boundaries between hypochondriasis and OCD are not at all clear. Hypochondriacal symptoms can of course occur in a variety of conditions; for example patients suffering from major depression may react with excessive concern to relatively minor bodily dysfunction. In OCD, obsessions about health are very common and can be very distressing for the individual, leading to time-consuming obsessional behaviours. Many clinicians assessing the compulsive checking and seeking of reassurance characteristic of the patient with hypochondriasis would justifiably conclude that they were observing symptoms of OCD. A separate diagnosis of hypochondriasis would not appear to be particularly useful.

Eating disorders

High rates of obsessional symptoms and obsessional features are reported in patients with anorexia nervosa and in those with bulimia. Traits such as rigidity and perfectionism are reported to be frequently found in anorexia nervosa, for example (Kaye et al 1993), and OCD symptoms are reported to be the most common comorbid symptoms apart from depressive symptoms (Rothenburg 1990). In patients diagnosed as OCD relatively high rates of eating disorders are also reported — between 10% and 17% anorexia nervosa and up to 20% bulimia (Rubenstein et al 1992).

Anorexia nervosa is frequently rather refractory to treatment but in bulimia and in some cases of anorexia nervosa the same treatments that are effective in OCD appear to be helpful (Wood 1993, Roberts and Lydiard 1994).

Impulse control disorders

Many disorders, which have been grouped loosely in the category of impulse control disorders, lack specific evidence of a link with OCD and much further research is needed. Thus pathological gambling, kleptomania, and other similar conditions are not considered here. Some self-injurious behaviour appears to have a more established link.

The compulsive nature of trichotillomania is recognized by those unfortunate individuals who have the compulsion persistently to pull their hair, often producing bald patches. There is some evidence that this condition responds to the same antiobsessional treatments as OCD (Swedo et al 1989) yet for many this response may be shortlived. Moreover there may be a response to serotonergic drugs in combination with a neuroleptic — a combination appropriate for Tourette's syndrome (Stein and Hollander 1993). There are similarities in the phenomenology of trichotillomania and Tourette's and it is possible that there is a common underlying neurological pathology. Other self-injurious behaviours such as compulsive skin picking or nail biting may also be related, though little investigation has been carried out.

The OCD spectrum

An attempt has been made to conceptualize this wide range of disorders on a continuum of compulsive to impulsive behaviour. In this scheme OCD and BDD would be seen as having risk-avoidance characteristics, and trichotillomania, compulsive gambling, and self-injurious behaviour would be seen as positioned at the impulsive risk-seeking end of the continuum. Much further research is needed to explore the relationship between OCD and the disorders that have been suggested may belong to an OCD spectrum.

There are two main approaches to the treatment of OCD, psychological treatment and pharmacological treatment. However, most clinicians endorse a combined approach.

The most characteristic feature of pharmacological treatments for OCD, and the most interesting because of the clues it gives as to the biological substrate of the disorder, is the specificity of response to drugs with potent serotonin reuptake blocking activity. The successful treatments for OCD are antidepressants but only those with potent effects on the serotonergic neurotransmitter system appear to have antiobsessional efficacy. OCD does not respond to antidepressants lacking serotonin reuptake blocking activity even though these are effective in depression. Nor do the depressive symptoms, which occur frequently with OCD, respond to antidepressants without serotonergic effects (Table 11).

Clomipramine

The first effective pharmacological treatment for OCD was clomipramine, whose antiobsessional properties were observed by Fernandez and Lopez-Ibor in 1967. Since then an impressive body of placebo-controlled studies, both small and very large, has produced remarkably consistent evidence of the effi-

Drug	Minimum effective dose		Dose
Clomipramine	Flexible dose studies		100–300 mg
Fluvoxamine	Flexible dose studies only		100–300 mg
Fluoxetine	20 mg (Tollefson et al 1994)		30–60 mg
Paroxetine	40 mg (Wheadon et al 1993)		40 mg
Sertraline	50 mg (Greist et al 1995c)		50–200 mg

Table 11
Medication with demonstrated efficacy in OCD.

cacy of this drug in treating OCD. Clomipramine has been shown to be effective in the treatment of OCD in children as well as in adults (Flament et al 1985, de Veaugh Geiss et al 1992) (Table 12).

When the effect of clomipramine on obsessional symptoms was first identified it was supposed that the improvement could be attributed to the general antidepressant action of the drug. If this were the case, patients with depression and OCD would be more likely to respond than those without marked depressive symptoms. However, it is clear that the antiobsessional effect was not mediated via an antidepressant effect since clomipramine has been shown to be effective in treating patients with OCD who did not have significant depressive symptoms compared with placebo (Montgomery 1980, Marks et al 1988). This is supported by analysis of studies where patients with marked depressive symptoms were not excluded, which shows that initial level of depressive symptoms does not influence the antiobsessional effect.

If the efficacy of the antiobsessional drugs were related to an antidepressant action, the full range of antidepressants would be expected to be effective. In fact the only drugs that have

Study	n	Design	Outcome
Montgomery 1980	14	Crossover CMI 75 mg	CMI>placebo 4 weeks
Thoren et al 1980b	16	Parallel CMI 150 mg	CMI>placebo 5 weeks
Marks et al 1980	40	Parallel CMI mean 183 mg	CMI>placebo 4 weeks
Insel et al 1983	12	Crossover CMI 100–300 mg	CMI>placebo 4–6 weeks
Flament et al 1985	19	Crossover CMI 141 mg	CMI>placebo 5 weeks
Mavissakalian et al 1985	12	Parallel CMI 100–300 mg	CMI>placebo 12 weeks
Marks et al 1988	37	Parallel CMI 125–157 mg plus exposure in both groups	CMI>placebo 8 weeks
de Veaugh Geiss et al 1989	241	Parallel CMI 100–300 mg	CMI>placebo 2–10 weeks
de Veaugh Geiss et al 1989	143	Parallel CMI 100–300 mg	CMI>placebo 2–10 weeks

Table 12
Placebo-controlled studies of clomipramine in OCD.

been shown clearly to be effective antiobsessional treatments are those with important serotonergic activity. Antidepressants lacking this property have not produced promising results. Neither nortriptyline nor desipramine, both selective inhibitors of noradrenaline, appears to be effective in OCD and positive antiobsessional effect could not be established for amitriptyline or imipramine.

The lack of antiobsessional efficacy of desipramine, which is an effective antidepressant that affects noradrenaline but lacks serotonin reuptake inhibiting properties, has been shown in a number of direct comparisons with SRIs. Comparison with clomipramine or the SSRIs fluvoxamine and sertraline showed the failure of desipramine in the treatment of OCD (Zohar and Insel 1987, Goodman et al 1990, Bisserbe et al 1997). It seems that the antiobsessional response in OCD is specific to the serotonergic activity identified with clomipramine and the SSRIs.

Selective serotonin reuptake inhibitors (SSRIs)

The perception that serotonin plays an important role in OCD makes the SSRIs an obvious potential treatment. These drugs, which lack important pharmacological activity on other systems, offer an effective treatment for OCD that is well tolerated and generally acceptable to patients.

The results of the placebo-controlled studies that have been carried out with the SSRIs have been consistently positive. Fluvoxamine, fluoxetine, paroxetine, and sertraline have all been shown in large placebo-controlled studies to be effective in the treatment of OCD and open studies reported on citalopram suggest that this SSRI is also effective.

Fluvoxamine

Five placebo-controlled studies have shown the efficacy of fluvoxamine, the earliest of the SSRIs to be investigated in OCD. Positive results were reported in a series of early, relatively small studies (Perse et al 1987, Goodman et al 1989, Cottraux et al 1990). In one of these studies (Cottraux et al 1990) behaviour therapy was given concomitantly, which should have made it more difficult to identify the significant advantage of fluvoxamine compared to placebo since behaviour therapy is a potentially effective therapy. Nevertheless the efficacy of fluvoxamine was seen in this study. Large multicentre studies have been carried out more recently and these have confirmed the antiobsessional efficacy of fluvoxamine. The significant therapeutic effect was seen from between four and six weeks onwards (Greist et al 1995d, Goodman et al 1996).

A high dose of fluvoxamine was used in all the studies, ranging between 200 mg and 300 mg per day. There are no studies that used multiple fixed doses that would have allowed the identification of the optimum dosage regime, so it is not possible to determine the preferred dose.

Fluoxetine

The evidence for the efficacy of fluoxetine is derived from three positive studies, which compared multiple fixed doses of fluoxetine and placebo. Doses of 20 mg, 40 mg, and 60 mg were compared with placebo in a relatively small eight-week study (Montgomery et al 1993) and two 13-week studies (Tollefson et al 1994). In the eight-week study, 40 mg and 60 mg a day were both effective compared to placebo whereas 20 mg a day was not, but in the 13-week study all three doses of fluoxetine were effective compared to placebo though the greatest response was seen in the group receiving the highest does (Tollefson et al 1994).

An analysis carried out on the pooled data from the studies showed that fluoxetine exerted its therapeutic effect on both aspects of OCD, the obsessional thoughts and the compulsions. This was seen in the significant advantage of fluoxetine measured on the total score of the YBOCS, the most frequently used severity scale for OCD, and on the separate subscales (Wood and Tollefson 1993).

Paroxetine

The efficacy of paroxetine compared to placebo has been established both in a fixed-dose study that compared 20 mg,

40 mg, and 60 mg and in flexible-dose studies (Wheadon et al 1993, Zohar and Judge 1996). In the 12-week fixed-dose placebo-controlled study, which was a large study (348 patients), paroxetine in doses of 40 mg and 60 mg was effective and significantly better than placebo but the 20 mg regime was not. The advantage was registered on both the obsessional and compulsion subscales of the YBOCS showing that, like other antiobessional drugs, paroxetine exerts its therapeutic effect on both aspects of OCD. There was no difference between paroxetine and clomipramine, included in this study as a reference control, except for an advantage for paroxetine in treating the depressive symptoms (Zohar and Judge 1996).

Sertraline

The antiobsessional efficacy of sertraline has been shown in placebo-controlled flexible-dose, fixed dose and long-term studies (Chouinard et al 1990; Kronig et al 1994; Greist et al 1995a; Greist et al 1995a and c; Rasmussen et al 1997). Both flexible dose studies, which investigated sertraline in doses from 50 to 200 mg, showed a significant advantage for sertraline compared with placebo. The 12-week fixed dose study that compared sertraline in dosages of 50 mg, 100 mg and 200 mg with placebo found a flat dose-efficacy response relationship. From these data it appears that sertraline is the exception among the SSRIs in not showing a significant dose–response relationship. However, fluoxetine may have a flat dose-efficacy response (Greist et al 1995a).

The efficacy of sertraline is also seen in a 16-week double-blind study in 168 patients with OCD which compared sertraline in a dose range of 50–200 mg per day with clomipramine (50–200 mg per day) (Bisserbe et al). In the intention to treat, last observation carried forward analysis, sertraline was significantly more effective than clomipramine, measured on the improvement in the YBOCS, the NIMH Global OC and Clinical Global Impression of severity. Sertraline was clearly better tolerated than clomipramine and this advantage was reflected in the significantly lower number of treatment discontinuations in the sertraline treated group (10.5%) compared with patients who received clomipramine (25.6%).

The significant advantage ($p < 0.02$) for sertraline compared with desipramine in treating OCD (Hoehn-Saric et al 1997) is in accord with the body of evidence indicating that antidepressants lacking potent serotonin reuptake inhibiting activity are not effective in OCD. This comparison of sertraline with desipramine, which was conducted in 159 patients suffering from OCD and major depression, was interesting because sertraline was significantly more effective not only on the obsessional symptoms, but also in alleviating depressive symptoms. Remission, defined as a score on the Hamilton Depression Scale of ≤ 7, was achieved by 40% of sertraline-treated patients compared with only 24% of desipramine-treated patients ($p < 0.05$).

Citalopram

Early open case studies suggested efficacy for citalopram in OCD. The preliminary results from a recently completed placebo-controlled study in acute treatment have shown this drug to be effective. Efficacy was seen at doses of 20 mg, 40 mg and 60 mg, although the effect appeared most convincing at 60 mg (Montgomery 1998).

Case reports of other SRIs

The consistency of the results from placebo-controlled studies showing the antiobsessional efficacy of SSRIs supports the view that this is a pharmacological class effect and that other members of the class are likely candidate treatments for OCD. Some positive results have been reported from open case studies with the SSRI citalopram, and a placebo-controlled trial has been carried out. The therapeutic benefit of venlafaxine, a drug which has serotonin reuptake blocking properties as well as an effect on noradrenegic receptors, has also been reported (Rauch et al 1998). There are no double-blind studies but its role in the treatment of OCD needs investigation.

Dose of antiobsessional drug

The response of OCD to clomipramine or SSRIs differs somewhat from the response seen in depression and there is a general consensus that higher doses are needed in OCD.

The perception that higher doses are needed in OCD may have arisen partly because of the nature of the response, which for the most part is slow and incremental over some weeks before maximum response is reached. If the dose is raised in this early period, as is customary in a flexible dosage regime, response may be attributed to a higher dose than was necessary.

There is evidence to support the efficacy of low doses of antiobsessional drugs in some patients, for example clomipramine 75 mg was effective in one study compared with placebo (Montgomery 1980) and a significant effect was seen at low doses of clomipramine in the early part of another study where the dose was titrated upwards at the start of the study (de Veaugh Geiss et al 1989). In general, however, the studies that have compared fixed doses have indicated that a better response may be obtained with higher doses of antiobsessional drugs. A dose–response relationship has been shown with paroxetine with an advantage for doses of 40 mg and 60 mg compared with 20 mg, which was not different from placebo (Wheadon et al 1993). Similarly with fluoxetine there is a trend towards a better response with the higher dose of 60 mg (Tollefson et al 1994). The only SSRI for which there is no apparent dose–response relationship is sertraline. With this drug doses of 50 mg and 200 mg were both significantly better than placebo with a much less marked effect seen on the 100 mg dose. However, the response appeared to be somewhat greater on the 200 mg dose. Although more studies are needed, at this point, and based on these data, it appears that sertraline is the exception among the SSRIs in not showing a significant dose relationship.

Overall the evidence supports the clinical view that higher doses of SRIs than used in depression are likely to produce a better therapeutic effect. Therefore if treatment is initiated at a lower dose patients need to be reviewed for a possible increase in the dose if response is unsatisfactory.

Side-effects of antiobsessional drugs

The apparent obligation to use higher doses complicates treatment for OCD since a greater level of side-effects can be expected. The need for well tolerated drugs becomes particularly important. The tolerability of medication is also an important issue for a condition such as OCD, which is a long-term disorder where patients will be required to take medication over very long periods of time. The issue of side-effects is an important one since poorly tolerated drugs are likely to reduce a patient's willingness to continue taking medication and this will have an adverse effect on his or her chance of improvement (Table 13).

Clomipramine

Clomipramine is not selective in its pharmacological action and its effects on other systems than serotonin carry a heavy side-effects burden. In common with other older tricyclic antidepressants clomipramine is associated with important anticholinergic action which gives rise to dry mouth, blurred vision,

SSRI	Clomipramine
Nausea	Blurred vision
Vomiting	Dry mouth
Transient nervousness	Constipation
Insomnia	Tachycardia
Sexual problems	Urinary retention or hesitancy
Drowsiness	Sedation
	Orthostatic hypotension

Table 13
Side-effects of antiobsessional medication.

constipation, etc. The usefulness of clomipramine is restricted because of its unwanted side-effects. The anticholinergic side-effects may be so unpleasant that many patients are unable to continue taking medication.

SSRIs

The SSRIs have characteristic transient and short-lived (one to three weeks) serotonergic side-effects, in particular nausea and increases in anxiety. Persistent side-effects include sexual impairments and headache. However, in general the side-effects are relatively mild and well tolerated by patients. This is important in the treatment of any disorder but may be critical in OCD since the patients need long-term treatment.

Analysis of large databases from studies in depressed patients has shown that significantly more patients withdraw from treatment with tricyclic antidepressants prematurely compared with serotonin reuptake inhibitors (Montgomery et al 1994, Anderson and Tomenson 1995, Montgomery and Kasper 1995). This holds true for OCD patients and they stand a better chance of continuing treatment with an SSRI. The better tolerability profile was reported for sertraline in a comparison with desipramine where the discontinuations for adverse events were only 2.6% for sertraline compared with 21% for desipramine (Hoehn-Saric et al 1997). This effect was also seen in a comparison of sertraline with clomipramine (Bisserbe et al 1997) in which the withdrawals due to adverse events were 26% in the clomipramine-treated patients, mostly occurring within the first month, compared with 11% in the sertraline-treated group.

First-line treatment

Since the efficacy of both clomipramine and the SSRIs has been established in placebo-controlled trials the question of choice of one agent over another arises. If one were clearly more effective than another, this would inform the choice of treatment. There have been suggestions that the antiobsessional effect of clomipramine is more potent than that of the SSRIs, a view encouraged by some meta-analyses of published trial results (Greist et al 1995b, Piccinelli et al 1995). These meta-analyses, which compare recent studies of SSRIs with studies conducted many years ago with clomipramine, may, however, be misleading. Over the years since clomipramine was introduced there have been considerable changes in the patients treated and the response that is achieved. The size of the response to drug treatment tends to be smaller in recent studies than in the early studies of clomipramine and the response to placebo greater. As the availability of effective treatments has become known, a much greater range of patients has come forward for treatment and patients with less severe illness in whom amelioration would not be expected to be dramatic have been included in studies. The early studies are more likely to have included the persistent, severe, and untreated patients who would be expected to have a greater improvement with treatment and lower response to placebo.

The direct head-to-head comparisons of SSRIs with clomipramine, which would provide a fairer estimate of relative efficacy, show that all these drugs appear to have similar levels of efficacy. No significant differences have been found between clomipramine and fluoxetine (Pigott et al 1990, Lopez-Ibor et al 1996), fluvoxamine (Smeraldi et al 1992, Freeman et al 1994, Koran et al 1996, Milanfranchi et al 1997), and paroxetine (Zohar and Judge 1996). In the comparison of paroxetine and clomipramine a better effect on depression was seen with paroxetine and in the sertraline and clomipramine comparison there was even an advantage for sertraline in the intention to treat analysis (Bisserbe et al 1997). Some of these head-to-head comparisons were small studies and others used doses which were possibly less than optimal, but overall the studies suggest that the SSRIs and clomipramine have similar levels of efficacy (Table 14).

Study	n	SSRI
Pigott et al 1990	11	Fluoxetine ≤ 80 mg
Lopez-Ibor et al 1996	55	Fluoxetine 40 mg
Smeraldi et al 1992	10	Fluvoxamine ≤ 200 mg
Freeman et al 1994	64	Fluvoxamine ≤ 200 mg
Koran et al 1996	79	Fluvoxamine 100–200 mg
Milanfranchi et al 1997	26	Fluvoxamine ≤ 300 mg
Zohar and Judge 1996	300	Paroxetine ≤ 60 mg
Bisserbe et al 1997	168	Sertraline ≤ 200 mg

Table 14
Comparisons of serotonin reuptake inhibitors with clomipramine.

The choice of first-line treatment therefore needs to be made on the basis of safety and acceptability. Here the balance favours the SSRIs, which seem to be better tolerated. In the direct comparison of clomipramine and SSRIs clomipramine was less well tolerated and in the larger studies the dropouts on clomipramine were seen to compromise its efficacy (Bisserbe et al 1996, Zohar and Judge 1996). As well as having fewer withdrawals due to side-effects, particularly anticholinergic side-effects, the SSRIs have a much improved safety profile compared with clomipramine. Clomipramine is associated with a substantially elevated level of convulsions, reported at 1.5–2% in the higher doses often used in OCD compared with 0.1–0.5% in higher doses of different SSRIs. Moreover clomipramine is associated with a higher level of cardiotoxicity, which is reflected in the higher rate of deaths from overdose.

Comparator	Result
Clomipramine ≤ 250 mg	No difference
Clomipramine ≤ 150 mg	No difference
Clomipramine ≤ 200 mg	No difference
Clomipramine ≤ 250 mg	No difference
Clomipramine 100–250 mg	No difference
Clomipramine ≤ 300 mg	No difference
Clomipramine ≤ 250 mg	No difference
Clomipramine ≤ 200 mg	No difference

On the basis of a risk–benefit assessment the first-choice treatment should be an SSRI.

Differences among SSRIs

There appears to be little to choose between the SSRIs. Although each clinician may have a particular favourite there are few comparator data to provide a rational basis for choice. Selection of an SSRI may need to be made on the basis of other drugs the patient might need to take and the possibility of drug interactions. Fluoxetine and paroxetine are potent inhibitors of P450 isoenzymes CYP 2D6 which metabolize commonly used drugs such as tricyclic antidepressants, antipsychotics, and beta blockers. Sertraline is only a weak inhibitor of CYP 2D6. Fluvoxamine inhibits CYP 1A2, which affects the metabolism of warfarin and the hydroxylation of tricyclic antidepressants, and CYP 3A4, which metabolizes benzodiazepines and some antiarrhythmics.

The very long half-life of fluoxetine and its active metabolite make it difficult to initiate a change in the drugs a patient is taking since five to six weeks are needed to wash the drug out, though a variable combination of new and old drug may sometimes be envisaged. The long half-life may, however, be an advantage if the individual is thought likely to discontinue high-dose treatment abruptly. Some discontinuation side-effects can be expected with all antidepressants if treatment is withdrawn suddenly, and the longer half-life of fluoxetine, which ensures a slower withdrawal, may reduce this risk.

Long-term treatment

Anti-obsessional drugs appear to be effective in short-term treatment in between 60% and 80% of patients. However the quality of response suggests the need for long-term treatment strategies. The characteristic response of OCD is a steady incremental improvement, which continues over many weeks and may require treatment measured in months. Although some patients may respond within the first few weeks of treatment, 15–20% of patients respond much later (Goodman et al 1989). It is therefore important that courses of treatment should be of adequate length.

Two important questions are, what happens if the antiobsessional drugs are discontinued — do the patients relapse? — and if the drugs are continued, do they maintain their efficacy during long-term treatment?

Early open retrospective follow-up of patients who had responded to pharmacological treatment indicated that the improvement in symptoms was maintained only as long as medication was continued and that relapse would occur rapidly if it was discontinued (Thoren et al 1980b). Even patients who have remained well during treatment for a mean period of one year may relapse when the medication is withdrawn (Pato et al 1988) and this effect applies to both clomipramine and the SSRIs (Pato et al 1990).

The benefit obtained by maintaining treatment with clomipramine for a year was reported by Katz et al (1990) and since then a number of long-term studies, some for periods of longer than a year, have shown that response to SSRIs is sustained if medication is continued.

One thorough placebo-substitution study has shown the efficacy of paroxetine in long-term treatment in preventing relapse. There was a higher relapse rate among patients who were discontinued double blind to placebo following six months' successful treatment with paroxetine than in those who continued active treatment (Dunbar et al 1995). Double-blind extension data following an acute treatment study showed that the efficacy of paroxetine is maintained during long-term treatment. The sustained effect of SSRIs in long-term treatment is also seen in the one- and two-year extension studies from acute treatment studies with sertraline (Greist et al 1995a,

Rasmussen et al 1997). The long-term efficacy of fluvoxamine was shown in a study design which should have made it difficult to demonstrate efficacy, since behaviour therapy, a potentially effective treatment, was given to both groups.

In the one-year placebo-controlled study of Greist et al (1995a) the rate of discontinuation for adverse experiences dropped from 10% on sertraline during the initial 12 weeks to 4% during the 40-week continuation period (placebo 6% and 5% respectively). Overall 75% of the patients who entered the long-term study completed the study, which is a very high rate. This contrasts with the studies of clomipramine where, while the drug is effective, in those who continued taking the drug the rate of dropout is very high (Katz et al 1990).

These long-term studies have provided an important insight into the gradual nature of the response in OCD. Small but important therapeutic gains continue to be made over many months in these studies in responders to acute treatment, who continued on an open basis on long-term treatment (Figure 4).

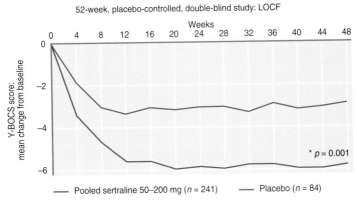

Figure 4
The gradual nature of response in OCD. Long-term efficacy of sertraline: Y-BOCS (Greist et al 1995a).

Medication for special groups

Children and adolescents

The onset of OCD is often in childhood or adolescence. It is important to recognize and treat OCD in these age groups. Once the diagnosis has been established medication can be considered, within the context of a combined behavioural and pharmacotherapeutic approach which involves the family.

A placebo-controlled, 11 weeks study demonstrated that clomipramine, a TCA with potent serotonin reuptake inhibitory properties, was effective in the treatment of adolescents (6–18 years) with OCD (Flament et al 1985). As might be expected the SSRIs also appear to be effective in young people (Riddle et al 1992).

The efficacy of sertraline for the treatment of OCD and depression in children and adolescents was suggested in an open study in 61 patients between the ages of 6 and 17 years (Alderman et al 1998). There were significant improvements in mean Children's Yale-Brown Obsessive Compulsive Scale, National Institute of Mental Health Global Obsessive Compulsive Scale (MIMH) and Clinical Global Impressions (CGI). Pharmacokinetic parameters were similar to those previously found in adults. The adult sertraline dosing regimen appeared suitable for use in children or adolescents. However, a lower starting dose of 25 mg/day was suggested to improve tolerability in children, particularly those with low body weight. In a further randomized double-blind, placebo-controlled study (March et al) 187 patients aged 6 to 17 years old were randomized to receive either sertraline or placebo for 12 weeks. Sertraline-treated patients exhibited significantly greater improvement than placebo-treated patients on the CY-BOCS, NIMH Global scale, Clinical Global Impression Scale-Improvement and Severity (CGI-I and CGI-S) scales. No clinically meaningful abnormalities were seen in vital signs, laboratory tests or electrocardiographic assessments in patients receiving sertraline.

Sertraline has a registered use in this population in the USA and in some European countries, although not in the UK.

The elderly

Age is no bar to treatment and effective antiobsessional medication is effective across the age range. Some caution will be needed in treating the elderly patient with OCD, first because of the physiological changes associated with ageing which affect the way the drugs are handled by the body and, secondly, because of the increased likelihood that the person will be taking medication for other concomitant physical conditions. Close attention needs to be paid to dosage, choice of medication, and the safety issues of treatment.

Other drugs

Clomipramine and the SSRIs are the accepted effective treatments for OCD with a strong body of evidence from placebo-controlled studies to support them. The results of studies of other drugs have not been encouraging.

A preliminary analysis suggested that mianserin was effective compared with placebo at four weeks (Jaskari 1980); one small study found an effect with clonazepam (Hewlett et al 1992), and another found some effect with L-tryptophan (Montgomery et al 1992). There is little evidence to support the use of monoamine oxidase inhibitors: clorgyline was less effective than clomipramine in one small study and in another no difference was found between phenelzine and clomipramine (Insel et al 1983, Vallejo et al 1992, Jenike et al 1997). The anxiolytic drug buspirone was not effective in open treatment although one small study did not find a difference between clomipramine and buspirone (Table 15). On the other hand, the augmentation of treatment with SSRIs or clomipramine with a number of other drugs may be helpful in certain subgroups of OCD (see the following chapter).

Study	n	Design	Outcome
Mianserin (MIAN) Jaskari 1980	40	CMI (150 mg) MIAN (60 mg) Placebo	Preliminary analysis only; ?MIAN > placebo (4 weeks)
Corgyline (CLOR) Insel et al 1983	23	Crossover CMI (100–300 mg) CLOR (30 mg)	CMI > CLOR (6 weeks)
L-tryptophan (TRP) Montgomery et al 1992	17	Crossover TRP (3 g) Placebo	?TRP > placebo ($p = 0.1$)
Trazodone (TRZ) Pigott et al 1992	17	TRZ (≤ 300 mg) Placebo	TRZ = placebo
Phenelzine (PHE) Vallejo et al 1992	26	CMI (≤ 225 mg) PHE (≤ 75 mg)	CMI = PHE (12 weeks)
Jenike et al 1997	41	PHE (60 mg) vs. placebo	
Buspirone (BUS) Pato et al 1991	18	BUS (60 mg) CMI (≤ 250 mg)	BUS = CMI
Clonazepam (CLO) Hewlett et al 1992	25	CLO (10 mg) CMI (250 mg) Placebo (diphenhydramine)	CLO > placebo CMI > placebo CLO = CMI (6 weeks)

CMI = clomipramine

Table 15
Double-blind comparative studies of other compounds in the treatment of OCD.

Summary

Response to pharmacological treatment follows a gradual course with small increments over many months. The anti-obsessional action appears to be specific to serotonergic medication and is directed to both obsessional thoughts and compulsive behaviours since patients in whom one or the other type of symptom predominates all respond. A greater effect of treatment with antiobsessional medication is registered in patients with more severe OCD compared with the milder cases. This is important, since behaviour therapy appears to be less appropriate for patients who are severely ill. However, only two thirds of the patients respond to serotonergic medication, emphasizing the importance of further research in this area.

Treatment-resistant OCD

Despite the significant progress that has been achieved in the treatment of OCD, 30–40% of OCD patients do not respond at all to treatment or respond poorly (Table 16). The problem of treatment resistance and its management is complicated by our lack of understanding of the underlying pathophysiology of OCD and the mechanisms by which different treatments produce their beneficial effects.

To a large degree we have to take an empirical, trial-and-error approach in treating resistant OCD since evidence from controlled studies is not available to support a recommendation for the various strategies that have been proposed. Pharmacological treatment for the treatment-resistant OCD patient can be divided into six stages during which unsuccessful pharmacological treatment with conventional antiobsessional agents can be followed by augmentation strategies, alternative primary agents or routes of administration, and finally by neurosurgery.

1 Initial treatment

The initial pharmacological treatment with one of the first-line therapies, clomipramine or an SSRI, should have been continued for sufficient time at an adequate dose before it is assumed that a patient is not responding to treatment.

- Inadequacy of trial
  - — duration too short?
  - — dose too low?
  - — impaired absorption/increased metabolism?
  - — noncompliance?
- Coexisting condition limits drug efficacy
- Incorrect diagnosis?
- Exogenous countertherapeutic influences
  - — family environment?
  - — antiexposure instructions?
- Underlying biological heterogeneity
  - — OCD as a syndrome with multiple aetiologies
- Search for putative subtypes

Goodman et al 1993

Table 16
Reasons for SRI refractoriness.

2 Change medication

If patients cannot tolerate adequate trials of SSRIs or do not respond to any of the SSRIs administered in the upper range of the relevant dose for at least 12 weeks at maximum dose, a trial of clomipramine at a dose of 200–300 mg/day for 12 weeks is recommended. Caution is needed if clomipramine is administered immediately following fluoxetine because the long half-life of fluoxetine and its inhibition of cytochrome P450 enzymes, which would increase the availability of clomipramine, dictate lower initial doses of clomipramine. Alternatively, if the patient has not responded to clomipramine, a move to SSRIs can be tried, although data regarding the efficacy of SSRIs in OCD patients who are nonresponders to clomipramine are scant.

3 Augmentation strategies

In the event of nonresponse the next approach can be to combine serotonergic therapies, for example the combination of clomipramine with an SSRI, or adding to clomipramine or an SSRI either a neuroleptic (fenfluramine, lithium, tryptophan) or buspirone. It is, however, very important to bear in mind the possible interaction between drugs when they are combined. For example, in the case of fluoxetine and clomipramine, the interaction between the two has been reported to increase the blood levels of tricyclics.

Neuroleptics

Some patients who do not respond to treatment are found to be also suffering from tic disorder. This subgroup of patients may in fact constitute a subtype of OCD. If a diagnosis of tic disorder accompanies that of OCD, the addition of small doses of dopamine blockers (ie neuroleptics) to the serotonergic drug has been shown to be associated with greater therapeutic response (McDougle et al 1990).

Lithium

Augmentation with lithium was not effective in the only double-blind placebo-controlled study of this combination (McDougle et al 1991). However, as some refractory patients may respond to lithium augmentation it could be tried in nonresponders. Augmentation may last for at least three weeks and lithium blood levels of 0.6–0.9 mEq/1 are desirable.

Fenfluramine

Fenfluramine, a serotonin releaser and reuptake inhibitor, has been associated with further decrease in OCD symptoms when combined with SSRIs in several open case reports although there are no double-blind controlled studies (Hollander et al

1990, Judd et al 1991). An adequate trial of fenfluramine augmentation should probably last at least 8 weeks at a dosage of 20–60 mg/day.

Buspirone

Although studies of buspirone alone in the treatment of OCD have generally yielded negative results, augmentation with buspirone might be considered as an option, as a few patients may benefit from the combination of buspirone with SSRIs (Markovitz et al 1990).

Tryptophan

There have been conflicting reports on the efficacy of L-tryptophan, the amino-acid precursor of serotonin, but augmentation may be a valid option for refractory patients. There were concerns about an association of tryptophan with eosinophilia myalgia syndrome but change in the manufacturing process has allowed it to be reintroduced. The recommended dose of tryptophan is 2–10 mg/day.

4 Alternative medication

Atypical neuroleptics

Although a therapeutic effect was reported in one case of treatment with clozapine, clozapine did not appear to be effective in 20 treatment-resistant OCD patients treated for 10 weeks (McDougle et al 1995a). Open treatment studies have reported an effect in alleviating OCD symptoms with risperidone (McDougle et al 1995b), but exacerbation of OCD after administration of risperidone has also been reported (Remington and Adams 1994).

Thyroid supplementation

Tri-iodothyronine has been reported to be efficacious in open trials as adjunctive agents to SRIs. However, the efficacy of this agent in OCD was not confirmed in a controlled study (Pigott et al 1991). The recommended dose of liothyronine is 25–50 µg/day.

Clonidine

Clonidine, an alpha-2 adrenergic agonist, has been reported to be effective in treating OCD symptoms in the context of Tourette's syndrome (Cohen et al 1980) and there are reports of improvement in typical OCD patients (Knesevich 1982, Hollander et al 1988). However, there are no controlled data to support the efficacy of this agent and the associated side-effects discourage its use for OCD patients.

Monoamine oxidase inhibitors (MAOIs)

Early studies did not support the antiobsessional efficacy of MAOIs (Insel et al 1983) though a recent study suggested that phenelzine might have an effect similar to clomipramine (Vallejo et al 1992). MAOIs might therefore be tried in refractory cases, especially where atypical depression and/or panic disorder are also present. Doses of phenelzine up to 90 mg/day for at least 10 weeks are proposed (Rauch and Jenike 1994). Caution is needed in switching between serotonin-reuptake inhibitors and an MAOI to allow a sufficient period of washout following discontinuation to avoid potentially dangerous interactions. This is particularly important in OCD patients, some of whom are hypersensitive to activation of their serotonergic system (Zohar 1996). For shorter half-life SSRIs (such as fluvoxamine and sertraline), the washout should be at least 2 weeks and with fluoxetine it should be even longer.

Intravenous clomipramine

The efficacy of intravenous clomipramine has been reported in a small number of patients with intractable OCD (Warneke 1989, Fallon et al 1992). Infusions are given daily for around 14 days with a maximum dose of 325 mg/day. It is unclear why intravenous clomipramine should be effective in cases where oral clomipramine was ineffective.

Clonazepam

Conflicting results have been reported on the efficacy of the benzodiazepine clonazepam, which has effects on the sero-tonergic system, but some reports suggest it may be helpful (Rauch and Jenike 1994).

5 Other possibilities

ECT

Efficacy for ECT (electroconvulsive therapy) was reported in 32 treatment-refractory OCD patients, assessed by retrospective chart review (Maletzky et al 1994). However, the evidence is not compelling since any effect of ECT may have been directed to the depression present in 40% of the patients and the method of assessing change in OCD was not efficient. ECT should probably be reserved for the symptomatic (antidepres-sive) treatment of severely depressed and suicidal OCD patients. It is possible that ECT might reverse the resistant state and allow antiobsessional drugs to regain efficacy.

Antiandrogen therapy

The antiandrogen cyproterone acetate has been reported by one group of researchers to alleviate OCD symptoms (Casas et al 1986) but this finding has not been replicated. Further investigation is warranted but the approach remains experimental.

6 Neurosurgery

When all other treatments have failed, some patients with OCD are so severely ill that neurosurgery is considered. Current operations include anterior cingulotomy, anterior capsulotomy, subcaudate tractotomy, and limbic leucotomy. These procedures are beneficial for some patients and are relatively safe. Controlled studies of neurosurgery are obviously difficult to perform but follow-up studies suggest that between 40% and 60% of refractory patients can benefit, either fully or partially, from neurosurgery. Some patients, for whom response to neurosurgery has been only partial, display a better response following neurosurgery to other treatment modalities that were previously ineffective (Figure 5).

Summary

Despite the significant progress that has been achieved in the treatment of OCD, 20–30% of patients are still treatment resistant. In the treatment of resistant cases it is important to maintain the patient's hope along with a step-by-step logical approach. Although the focus here has been on the pharmacological approach, combination of pharmacological treatment with cognitive and behavioural therapy as well comprehensive family intervention is likely to give the best chance of achieving a good response (Table 17).

Stage 1		SSRI or clomipramine
	Comorbid Tic + OCD	Add neuroleptic
Stage 2	Switching	SSRI ↔ clomipramine
Stage 3	Augmenting	Lithium, risperidone, hormone, tryptophan, buspirone, trazodone
Stage 4	Other treatments	Intravenous clomipramine, MAOI, clonidine, clonazepam, atypical neuroleptics
Stage 5		ECT
Stage 6		Psychosurgery

Figure 5
Treatment of resistant OCD: behaviour therapy, when it becomes possible, is recommended as an integral part of treatment.

Treatment

- Switching to another potent SRI
- Combination treatments: add another agent (drug or behavioural therapy) to the SRI
- Novel and experimental drug treatments
- Nonpharmacologic biological approaches

Goodman et al 1993

Table 17
Treatment strategies for SRI-resistant OCD.

Psychological approaches to treatment

While pharmacotherapy tries to modify neurotransmitters in order to bring about amelioration of symptoms, behaviour therapy and cognitive therapy strive to change patterns of behaviour or attitudes and ways of interpreting events and thereby reduce distressing thoughts and dysfunctional behaviours.

The rationale for psychological treatments was based on the behavioural or learning theory of OCD. Briefly this suggests that OCD is a problem of learnt maladaptive behaviours. Obsessions are stimuli that have acquired an anxiety-evoking property and the individual undertakes compulsions to reduce anxiety. The reduction in anxiety is rewarding and the likelihood of further compulsive behaviour is increased.

Psychological treatments address the maladaptive behaviours directly, seeking to unlearn the faulty behaviours. There are problems with this account since few OCD patients report unpleasant events that triggered the original obsessions and many report that rather than serving to reduce anxiety, the compulsive behaviours actually increase it. Others report that anxiety does not describe the discomfort they suffer. Nevertheless the therapies, both behavioural and cognitive, that have been developed from this theoretical basis appear to be effective in the treatment of OCD.

Behaviour therapy

Behaviour therapy involves the OCD patient learning to exert self-restraint when faced by the situations which have been provoking compulsive behaviours. The use of behavioural techniques in OCD has a long history and was first suggested by Janet, who noted that the enforced discipline associated with joining the army or clergy brought about a reduction in obsessions and compulsions in individuals with OCD. He proposed a form of behaviour therapy that emphasized *exposure* to the feared stimulus. However, the modern age of effective behaviour therapy for OCD began with Meyer's reports that sustained *prevention of anxiety-reducing rituals* could also lead to a reduction in obsessions (Meyer 1996).

Exposure and response prevention

It is recognized that exposure is the essential feature of a behavioural treatment programme, but exposure combined with response prevention is the most widely recognized psychological treatment for OCD and has been the most thoroughly researched. Patients following a course of exposure and response prevention learn to expose themselves to those distressing activities or situations which they avoid, and resist their compulsions. The individual is forced to experience and learn to tolerate the discomfort of the feared situation without the relief of anxiety-reduction rituals. As the procedure is repeated it is thought that the anxiety response habituates — a phenomenon that may occur via fatigue associated with the continual excitation of sensory neurones. The habituation of the anxiety renders the anxiety-reducing rituals redundant and it is postulated that any future performance of the rituals is not rewarding and consequently they drop away.

The essentials of behaviour therapy

Although there are many variations in behavioural treatment programmes, which are tailored to fit individual patients, some general principles can be outlined.

Behavioural assessment (mapping)

The patient is helped to identify the triggers for the obsessions and compulsions and these are then ordered into a hierarchy from the most to the least distressing. Early behavioural approaches began with exposure to the least troublesome situations and, as the patient learnt to confront these, the more difficult situations were addressed. This hierarchical approach is adopted by some therapists though others take the approach of addressing the more serious problems earlier.

Specific rules of exposure

The patient and therapist agree together at what point in the hierarchy of problem situations the patient is able to start the exposure treatment. The patient is required to expose him or herself to a specific situation whilst agreeing not to engage in the usual rituals. For example, a patient with washing rituals might be asked to handle a dirty item (in vivo exposure) and not to wash afterwards (response prevention). Since many patients with this problem avoid touching clean items to avoid contamination, the instruction would also be given that they should not avoid touching clean objects, in other words not to exercise avoidance whilst 'contaminated'. An important element in the programme is that reassurance does not reduce the impact of the exposure. The patient gradually progresses from less intense to more prolonged exposure.

A key element in exposure therapy is that the patient experiences the full discomfort he or she would usually feel in the discomfort-provoking situation. Many patients are adept at avoiding these feared situations and find ways of minimizing the exposure, for example by brief contact, by touching with specific designated parts of their body, or by practising a mental neutralizing ritual. Skill is needed to identify these and to discuss with the patient their role in frustrating therapy.

Behaviour therapy for different types of OCD

Although most treatment programmes include both exposure and response prevention it has been suggested that different elements are more important for different types of obsessional behaviour. Thus exposure may be important for patients where there is a marked phobic profile, as in those with a fear of contamination and washing compulsions. Conversely, in patients with checking rituals, which seems to be a more complicated phenomenon involving associated doubt, guilt, and a heightened sense of responsibility, response prevention might be the most important aspect of the treatment (Rachman and Hodgson 1980).

Pure obsessionals

Most OCD sufferers have both obsessions and compulsions but some 2% of individuals appear to have no visible behavioural rituals or even mental rituals. These are patients to whom it is much more difficult to apply behavioural techniques, since it is obviously not easy to maximize exposure to covert obsessional phenomena. One widely used technique has been thought-stopping, where a command is used to terminate the unwanted thought — in the first instance given by the therapist and later by the patient. This approach may be more successful if the thought-stopping is applied to anxiety-provoking thoughts (Kirk 1983). In satiation or habituation training, patients are helped to focus on their distressing thoughts for prolonged periods (Rachman 1976, Emmelkamp and Kwee 1977). Spoken reminders, exposure to stimuli that provoke the thoughts, or written repetition of the thought or repetition on audiotape can all be used to direct and intensity the exposure.

Efficacy of behaviour therapy

A considerable body of studies has reported on the efficacy of behaviour therapy in OCD (reviewed Foa et al 1985), though most of these investigations were uncontrolled. It is of course difficult to find an adequate neutral control against which to test the effect of behaviour therapy, and preserving the blindness to treatment both in patients and the assessors presents a considerable problem. The early controlled studies, which used relaxation therapy as a control, were small, of short duration, and treatment was not always properly randomized (Roper et al 1975, Marks et al 1975, 1980).

The positive results of later studies that used antiexposure therapy as a control (Marks et al 1988) are limited by the possibility that antiexposure may not be a neutral control and may serve to make patients worse. A second study that used antiexposure (Cottraux et al 1990) did not find a significant difference between exposure and antiexposure treatments. This study combined behavioural treatment with pharmacotherapy and showed the efficacy of fluvoxamine compared with placebo. Since exposure therapy was given to both drug-treated and placebo-treated patients, if it were a powerful treatment one might have expected any drug placebo difference to be obscured. In view of the significant advantage for fluvoxamine, the SSRI examined in this study, it seems likely that the behaviour therapy combined with the SSRI exerted an additive antiobsessional effect.

A welcome recent study has addressed the problem of an appropriate control or behaviour therapy. In this study, 18 patients were treated with either exposure with response prevention or a general anxiety management intervention. Both treatments were applied in similar ways taking up the same amount of therapist and homework time. There was a significant advantage for behaviour therapy, which supports the clinical view that behaviour therapy is an effective form of treatment (Lindsay et al 1997).

A number of meta-analyses of studies have been published which assert that behaviour therapy has comparable or even greater improvement measured on the Y-BOCS scale in comparison to treatment with potent serotonin reuptake inhibitors (Table 18). The findings are, however, difficult to interpret

Study references	Design	Outcome
Marks et al 1975 includes: Rachman et al 1971, 1973, Hodgson et al 1972	Relaxation then exposure; not randomised; $n = 15$ vs $n = 20$; duration 3 weeks	Significant advantage for exposure doubtful; insufficient data
Roper et al 1975	Exposure or relaxation, then exposure; $n = 5$ vs $n = 5$ vs $n = 10$; duration 2–3 weeks	Significant advantage for exposure doubtful; insufficient data
Marks et al 1980	Exposure + placebo vs relaxation + placebo; $n = 10$ vs $n = 10$; duration 3 weeks	No group difference reported
Marks et al 1988	Exposure + CMI vs antiexposure + CMI; n - 12 vs n - 11; duration 17 weeks	?Exposure significantly better than antiexposure
Cottraux et al 1990	Exposure + fluvoxamine vs antiexposure + fluvoxaine; $n = 20$ vs $n = 20$; duration 24 weeks	Exposure not significantly different from antiexposure
Lindsay et al 1997	Exposure + response prevention vs general anxiety management; $n = 9$ vs 9; duration 3 weeks	Exposure and response prevention significantly better than anxiety management
	CMI = clomipramine	

Table 18
Controlled studies of behaviour therapy in OCD.

owing to the widely differing methodologies used, the difficulty of comparing placebo-controlled double studies of pharmacotherapy with inadequately controlled studies of psychological treatment, and the problem of how to weight the results of open studies (Christensen et al 1987, Cox et al 1993, van Balkom et al 1994).

Maintenance of response

Follow-up studies have claimed that patients who have been treated with behaviour therapy maintain their gains for from two to six years. However, these rates of improvement are likely to have been overestimated since, in clinical practice, many patients refuse to enter behavioural programmes and the dropout from treatment is substantial. Expansive claims have been made for the enduring efficacy after treatment of behaviour therapy though these claims have generally been made on the basis of uncontrolled follow-up. A review of the response in 273 patients treated in open trials of behaviour therapy reported that 51% of patients were cured or much improved — defined as having a greater than 70% reduction in symptoms (Foa et al 1985). At follow-up, 76% of these patients had continued their response and maintained a symptom reduction of at least 60%.

The controlled studies of long-term efficacy are much less optimistic. In the only controlled study of relapse prevention in 18 patients, a relapse rate of 66% within six months was observed for those who discontinued behaviour therapy compared with a relapse rate of 25% measured on the YBOCS in those who continued treatment (Hiss et al 1994). The study was well designed, with responders to three weeks' acute treatment with intensive exposure and response prevention being randomly assigned to receive either continued active treatment with behaviour therapy or deep muscle relaxation therapy given as the control for six months.

These results from a carefully controlled study contrast sharply with the open reports, as they often do, and made it clear that claims for an enduring effect of behavioural treatments are unrealistic. The relapse rate observed on continued behavioural treatment of 25% is in line with the relapse rate seen within a relapse prevention study with the SSRI paroxetine (39%). The relapse rate on discontinuation of behaviour therapy to relaxation treatment was 66% compared with 60% after discontinuing paroxetine to placebo (Dunbar et al 1995).

These results, although they come from controlled investigations using very different methodologies and populations, emphasize the need for continued treatment in OCD whether by behaviour therapy or pharmacotherapy in order to reduce the chance of the relapse of OCD.

It appears that behaviour therapy needs to be continued or the gains will be largely lost. Relapse-prevention techniques after intensive behaviour therapy need to be implemented to help patients persist with the behavioural approaches to their problems they have learnt. The success of this approach was reported by Hiss and colleagues (1994) and also by McKay and colleagues (1996), who developed a relapse-prevention programme of six months' duration although they found that depressive symptoms increased in the follow-up period.

Cognitive therapy

Cognitive therapy was developed originally by Aaron T Beck (1976), who viewed compulsions as attempts to allay excessive doubts. Anxiety was provoked not by a particular situation or thought but by the consequences of the situation or thought. It has also been suggested that normal intrusive thoughts become obsessional if the person thinks the thought is potentially harmful and takes the responsibility for causing this harm. Anxiety results and neutralizing responses are developed to reduce the anxiety (Salkovskis 1985).

Cognitive therapeutic techniques aim to have a direct effect in changing beliefs and thoughts — the way that patients perceive things. The treatment involves identifying 'inaccurate thoughts' or dysfunctional ways of thinking and showing the link between these thinking patterns and behaviours. Patients are taught to challenge the unhelpful thoughts and to replace them with other ways of thinking. Behavioural experiments are often used to test the validity of the thoughts that have been identified as unhelpful to help the replacement process.

The main focus of cognitive therapy in OCD has been the modification of abnormal risk assessment, which overestimates the probability of danger, and exaggerated responsibility feelings, which overestimate the consequences of a 'danger'. Patients are encouraged to arrive at a corrective framework of the actual probability of feared events within which they can examine their own assessments of risk. A similar approach is adopted for exaggerated responsibility with patients being encouraged to assess the contribution of all factors to an event in order to arrive at the modesty of the patient's own contribution to a feared situation.

The number of patients treated in controlled studies of cognitive therapy in OCD is still very small and assessments of its efficacy must therefore be cautious. Some investigators have reported an advantage for cognitive therapy compared with behaviour therapy (van Oppen et al 1995) whilst others found it to be effective though not more so than behaviour therapy (Emmelkamp et al 1988). Further research to establish the exact role of cognitive therapy is needed.

Combined behavioural and pharmacotherapy

Behavioural treatments, with or without cognitive restructuring, require high levels of motivation and commitment from the individual in order to obtain benefit. Motivation is often impaired by the severity of the disorder so that those benefiting from behaviour therapy tend to be less severe than those benefiting from antiobsessional medication. Few studies have examined the efficacy of combining the two treatment modalities. The study of Marks et al (1988) and Cotteaux et al (1990) showed that pharmacotherapy was able to give significant extra efficacy compared to placebo despite the concomitant behaviour therapy given to both groups. This supports the widespread belief that the treatments are additive in their effects and that the best response will come from using behavioural techniques alongside antiobsessional pharmacotherapy.

Recognizing OCD

The first problem in the management of OCD is the identification of those with the disorder. Sufferers are often secretive about the nature of their problem; they are embarrassed and fear ridicule. They may be prepared to discuss depression, anxiety, or somatic features more readily than their obsessions. However, those with OCD recognize that their obsessions and compulsions are not normal and a direct question about obsessions and rituals is answered for the most part with relief and the diagnosis can be established.

Choice of treatment

There are two established first-line modalities of treatment: the serotonergic reuptake inhibitors and behavioural treatments. The choice will depend on individual preference and available resources. Approximately 25% of OCD sufferers refuse behaviour therapy, and roughly the same proportion refuse medication.

Patients suffering from more severe OCD may well lack the motivation to participate in a behavioural treatment. Or they think they will be unable to withstand the stress involved in exposure and response prevention. For these patients treatment with a serotonin reuptake inhibitor would be more appropriate in the first instance. Other patients may have obsessional concerns about not taking drugs and for them behavioural treatments are the obvious choice.

It is the experience of most clinicians that the best treatment responses are seen when a combination of medication and behavioural treatments is used. Several studies have shown that the combination of pharmacotherapy and behaviour therapy, each an independently effective treatment for OCD, can be more effective than either treatment alone. Medication can improve compliance with behaviour therapy and behaviour therapy may help maintain the gains made during pharmacological treatment.

It may be necessary with individual patients to start with one or other treatment approach and move to a combination later. Patients whose treatment begins with antiobsessional drugs may be persuaded to accept a behavioural programme as their condition improves and their motivation strengthens. Likewise those patients whose obsessions include a fear of drug treatment may be persuaded by an incremental cognitive behavioural programme to initiate drug treatment.

Choice of medication

The choice between different drugs is based on efficacy and tolerability. It appears from the direct comparisons between the individual SSRIs and clomipramine that there is no difference in efficacy. However, there are substantial side-effect problems and serious adverse drug reactions reported with clomipramine.

It is usual to begin with the equally effective but better tolerated SSRIs. Evidence is lacking to support the choice of one of these drugs over another, which seem to have the same level of efficacy as each other. For reasons that are difficult to understand, indivdual patients may respond to one SSRI and not another. It is entirely reasonable therefore to switch between drugs of this class to obtain extra efficacy and possibly improved tolerability for the individual patient.

Clomipramine is generally reserved for those cases that do not respond to SSRIs because it carries a heavy side-effect burden that some patients find difficult to tolerate.

Experience has shown that response in some patients may not occur on the lower doses of antiobsessional drugs and a higher dose may be needed. Response to treatment is, however, slow and it is not possible to say whether a drug has not had some effect until after two or three months' treatment. Further improvement is often reported as much as six months or a year later.

Behaviour therapy and cognitive therapy

There are differences of opinion about the relative efficacy of behavioural or cognitive therapy. Both forms of psychological treatment seem to be effective and the choice may well depend on the availability and expertise of the particular practitioner.

One of the problems of behavioral treatments is the high level of motivation required of the patient and another is the time needed to maximize treatment. Motivation may be improved if patients are given information on what is involved in treatment and on likely outcome, or access to patients who have responded well to treatment.

The cost of behavioural treatments of sufficient length is high and this type of treatment may not be accessible to many patients because of lack of resources. Economic pressures have encouraged interest in the development of self-applied behavioural treatments, which can take over after initial therapist-directed treatment. This is a natural progression since behavioural treatment programmes lay emphasis on 'homework' between therapist-led sessions. The more the sufferer can take over the treatment from the therapist the more likely it is that the gains will persist.

Partial and poor response

Despite the efficacy of both behavioural and pharmacological treatments the quality of response seen is often less than optimal with a residuum of obsessional thoughts and behaviours which interfere to a greater or lesser extent with the functions of the sufferer. The proportion of partial responders to these treatments is unfortunately high and the proportion of those who are resistant to treatment is uncomfortable.

Various devices have been recommended in the case of those with resistant OCD but the first step should be the redoubling of the primary treatment: increasing the dose of SSRI, checking compliance, and increasing frequency and focus of behavioural treatments. Thereafter the range of potential extra treatments outlined in this chapter would need to be tried.

Information for patients

Until recently knowledge about OCD was not widespread and even now many medical practitioners as well as the public lack information about the disorder. To some extent this explains why there is often a very long delay between the appearance of troublesome symptoms of OCD and a sufferer seeking medical help. Often the individual has been unaware that effective treatments are available for the condition, which he or she has kept hidden sometimes even from his or her close family. The knowledge that OCD is a treatable condition suffered by millions of people worldwide often brings considerable relief to the sufferer.

Treatment is more likely to succeed in the context of a positive therapeutic relationship. Patients need information about the condition and about the treatments available in order to make an informed choice. Time is needed to detect the OCD, to discuss the particular problems of the patient, and to share the decision on treatment with the patient.

Information on what to expect from treatment is an essential element. This includes likely side-effects whether from drug treatment or the increase in anxiety engendered by behavioural treatments.

It is important that the expectations of patients are realistic and they need to be reassured that, although response may be slow, they should not be discouraged as it does continue with small increments over months. Patients who respond to treatment are often left with substantial residual symptoms and they need to know that the improvement achieved is such that it translates into far more important improvements in function and quality of life.

Family support

OCD is a disorder that often interferes not only with the life of the sufferer but also with the lives of those close to him or her. Relatives and friends of sufferers need to be drawn in on the support and information network. They need information on OCD, the symptoms, and the treatments in order to understand that this is a treatable disorder. Sometimes relatives feel that the OCD must somehow be their fault and they need to be reassured.

Families and friends can provide a great deal of support to the sufferer in making him or her feel less isolated, in his or her decision to seek professional help, and in his or her determination to recover. Encouragement and appreciation of small gains made provide positive help. However, those who care for the sufferer need to be well informed about the treatment programme and the need to avoid helping with the obsessional behaviours, or providing counterproductive reassurance, or adapting their way of doing things to accommodate the obsessions and rituals of the sufferer.

Self-help

Patients and their families can gain considerable support and help from consumer organizations, of which there are an increasing number (see the Appendix). The range of activities varies but an important feature they share is the contact they provide with others in similar situations. They are also a source of information on OCD, on the available treatments, how to reach treatment, useful books, self-help groups, etc.

Many OCD patients find benefit in joining a self-help group, for contact, information, but also for support in persisting with treatment programmes.

The number of self-help books to guide sufferers through their own behavioural treatment programme is increasing and those with milder OCD may find these particularly helpful. Similar initiatives with interactive computer programs are also being developed and are found to be helpful.

Common questions about OCD

Q How do I know if I really have OCD?

A You have OCD if you are carrying out behaviours excessively that you suspect may be OCD symptoms; or you wish you could do less — less washing, less checking, less ordering, less obsessed with aggressive, somatic, or sexual thoughts; or if the obsession and or compulsion interferes with your activities. A formal way to think about whether you suffer from OCD is if the total sum of the obsessions and compulsions takes more than an hour a day. If you are not quite sure about whether or not you have OCD the best advice is to share your concern with an expert.

Q How can I get family members to understand what I am going through?

A Your physician may be willing to talk with your family members and explain that OCD is a real disorder responding to appropriate treatment; that it does not mean that you are weak or doing things in order to annoy. Some consumer organizations such as the Obsessive Compulsive Disorder Foundation in the USA or Obsessive Action in the UK produce leaflets which explain the condition to family members and what they can do to help.

Q What can I do about my depression? Is it part of OCD?

A More than two thirds of OCD patients suffer from depression from time to time and it seems to be part of OCD. Depressive symptoms are often found as part of OCD and respond well to antiobsessional medication. The depression associated with OCD does not tend to respond to conventional antidepressants that do not have a specific antiobsessional effect nor is it thought to respond well to behaviour therapy.

Q I feel guilty about everything. What can I do about it?

A Some people's OCD comes out in the form of obsessional guilt which is out of proportion to the possible cause and has all the features of obsessional thoughts, coming back again and again in spite of reassurance. Like any other obsessional thought it should respond to appropriate treatment from an expert. If you are taking part in a self-help group it might help to bring this up and find out how fellow sufferers react.

Q Are people with OCD crazy?

A Part of the definition of OCD is that the sufferers are well aware of the excessive or unreasonable nature of their ritual or obsession. In all other areas of life the individual is functioning perfectly well. Those with OCD do not become psychotic, do not lose the proper interpretation of real events, but suffer from a specific limited problem. It is as if their assessment of risk is affected and they consider very remote possibilities as something they should be extremely worried about. The disorder is better understood nowadays, there is treatment, and sufferers are not crazy.

Q Is there a particular personality type associated with OCD?

A The consensus is that no particular personality type is associated with OCD. It might be thought that a patient who tends to be very meticulous, pedantic, overconscientious, or who finds it difficult to make decisions is more likely to get OCD. However, formal studies have not found this to be the case.

Q Is OCD made worse by stress?

A Everything gets worse in times of stress and OCD symptoms may appear to worsen too. OCD is not directly related to stress but may worsen at such moments, much as hypertension or asthma gets worse in times of stress. Some women complain of worsening before or during menstruation; other people experience worsening at moments like starting a new job, or doing examinations. Stress itself cannot be treated and is inevitable in life. The OCD, however, can be treated.

Q Is there something wrong with the brain of people with OCD?

A Progress in psychiatry in the last decade has led to the use of imaging techniques to examine brain activity. As a result we know there are specific changes in the brain of OCD patients as compared to people without OCD or to depressed patients. The changes relate to hyperactivity of the basal ganglia and prefrontal areas in the brain, which normalizes as the patient responds to treatment, whether the intervention is medication or behavioural.

Q What causes OCD?

A There are several hypotheses regarding the cause of OCD. The leading contender suggests abnormalities in a subset of the serotonergic system that might be genetic, secondary to inflammatory processes, secondary to trauma events, or some other unknown cause. Other investigators think that the dopaminergic system is implicated in OCD as well. The increased prevalence of OCD in pregnancy suggests a role for the hormones. There are some data that point to the possible involvement of an autoimmune mechanism. Behavioural therapists believe that OCD is a maladaptive learnt behaviour and cognitive psychologists suggest OCD arises in an individual who has adopted the 'wrong' brain script for interpreting events. Probably there are different subtypes of OCD, and more than one cause to this intriguing disorder.

Q What is the best treatment?

A There are two approaches to treatment, working on different principles, and both seem to work well. Behaviour therapy, with or without a cognitive component, requires considerable motivation and application on the part of the sufferer. Anti-obsessional drugs are seen to work on both obsessions and rituals and to deal with concomitant depression. In the experience of most experts behavioural and drug treatments combine well to produce the best treatment.

Q Does behaviour therapy work if I have more than one symptom?

A Usually behaviour therapy takes a hierarchical approach starting with the lighter problems and going on to those that are more difficult. Most people have more than one symptom.

Q How do I find out about the nearest specialist?

A Your GP is your first source of help. Consumer groups that aim to increase awareness of OCD may be able to make suggestions. The Internet also carries information on OCD.

Q How do I know if I need a therapist or just a self-help book?

A Several self-help books have been published in the last few years regarding behaviour therapy of OCD. Most of them might be helpful if combined with professional guidance. You would be well advised to talk first with an expert to be sure that your problems are indeed OCD and to discuss the treatment options. The use of self-help books is one of the options and can be part of a comprehensive professional treatment plan.

Q What kind of medication helps OCD symptoms?

A The medications that are effective in treating OCD have a specific profile affecting the serotonergic system (see earlier in this book for names and doses).

Q Are there side-effects?

A Every effective medication has some side-effects. It might be of interest for you to know that even sugar pills have side-effects. The new generation of antiobsessive medications (SSRIs) are generally well tolerated but some patients may have nausea or vomiting; others might have headache, drowsiness, insomnia, decrease in their libido, and/or ability to achieve orgasm, initially weight loss and sometimes weight gain later on. However, most of the side-effects will disappear after a few weeks of treatment. In most cases the only side-effects that may persist are the sexual side-effects and headache. The side-effects disappear when the drug is discontinued.

Q How long does it take before medication works?

A The way antiobsessional medication works probably relates to changes in the sensitivity of certain serotonergic receptors. These changes are brought about via feedback mechanisms and it therefore takes a long time (up to 12 weeks) before the antiobsessional medication works. This unfortunately means that, at the start of treatment, side-effects may be experienced but no obvious therapeutic benefit. People taking antiobsessional medication need to be aware that they will not experience any immediate effect such as we get, for example, from a painkiller, and that they need to persist with medication. By the same token it takes a few weeks after stopping the medication before there is exacerbation of OCD symptoms. We need to be aware that this therapeutic gap exists both after initiation and after stopping treatment.

Q Why do these drugs help?

A The medication probably helps by decreasing the sensitivity of the serotonergic receptors in OCD patients. The clinical manifestation of these changes is the increased ability of the individual to resist the obsessions and compulsions and a reduction in intensity of the obsession or compulsion.

Q Will I have to take antiobsessional medication for ever?

A The current knowledge about the usefulness of medication in this disorder has been gathered since 1980. We do not know how long it is necessary to continue with antiobsessional medication but we do know that if medication is stopped the symptoms very often recur. After a year your doctor might suggest attempting a very gradual reduction in the dose. Some people may be able to stop their antiobsessional medication after several years but others will need medication for longer.

Q How do I know if I am on the right dose of medication?

A The 'right' dose of a medication is the lowest dose where you feel benefit with the least side-effects. When treatment is started the dose of medication you are given might be somewhat higher than the dose usually recommended for depression. For example, if fluoxetine is prescribed you might be given 40–60 mg for OCD; paroxetine 40 mg, sertraline 50–200 mg, clomipramine 250 mg, fluvoxamine 250 mg. When you have improved, your doctor will probably suggest that you continue to take medication to keep you well. Your physician may, after a year or 18 months, suggest trying a lower dose and may reduce the dose in small increments of, for example, 25 mg reduction of paroxetine every six weeks, 50 mg sertraline or 50 mg fluvoxamine every six weeks. If by the end of the six weeks you have not had any worsening of symptoms your physician may suggest reducing the dose further, always watching carefully in case there is any exacerbation of your OCD.

Q What are the long-term consequences of drugs?

A All the antiobsessional drugs have been widely used as antidepressants and their long-term consequences closely monitored. The SSRIs have proved to be particularly safe and effective in the long term. So far it has been estimated that some 80 million people have taken these drugs world-wide over many years without any long-term concerns arising.

Q Can I get pregnant while taking the drugs?

A Doctors are cautious and they will all recommend that you avoid taking any drugs while you are trying to get pregnant or during the first three months of pregnancy. However, some people have become pregnant while taking SSRIs and follow-up studies claim that there is no evidence of elevated risk of problems. This is, however, a matter which must be discussed with your physician.

Q Do I need additional treatment to medication?

A It is quite clear that exposure is an important factor in the therapeutic process. Patients who are treated with medication are encouraged to capitalize on the therapeutic effect of the medication through exposure, by reducing the avoidance, by stopping the rituals that were originally attached to the obsession. Thus the treatment consists of the medication plus behavioural homework.

Q What therapy is best if I have only obsessional thoughts, not behaviours?

A OCD is unique in having a very specific response to medication, which affects the serotonergic system. In several studies it was found that the antiobsessive effect of medication is effective both for the obsessional thoughts and for the compulsions, the behavioural part of the disorder. Most of the data regarding behaviour therapy concern the behavioural part of the disorder but a good result may be obtained with certain types of behavioural techniques in patients who have obsessions alone. A combination of antiobsessional medication with 'thought-stopping' techniques might be helpful for this particular form of OCD.

Q Does hypnotherapy work?

A To be sure that a therapy works we would like to have scientific data showing that any effect is indeed attributable to the intervention. The usual way is to compare a treatment with a neutral control where preferably neither the physician nor the patient knows which treatment they are receiving, or where independent raters assess response. Unfortunately there are no data of this type regarding hypnotherapy in treating OCD. All we can say at this point is that it probably will not cause harm if carried out by a competent hypnotherapist but there is no evidence to suggest it is helpful.

Q Is there an association between allergies and OCD?

A There are currently no data to suggest an association between allergies and OCD. There are some very preliminary reports that suggest that in certain autoimmune disorders such as Sydenham's chorea there might be an increased prevalence of OCD which could be related to the development of antibodies to an area in the brain implicated in OCD, such as the caudate nuclei.

Q If OCD is caused by a chemical imbalance in the brain, how can therapy work?

A If we are afraid of something there is a definite physical change: we become pale, our pulse is increased, blood pressure goes up. The concept that psychological changes are associated with definite physical changes is well established. The principle of behaviour therapy is to change the way a patient responds by exposing the patient to what is most feared and preventing the usual obsessional response from being carried out. This is in a sense changing the wiring (in the brain). Studies that look at the activity of the brain before and after successful behavioural intervention have found definite changes.

Q No sooner do I get rid of one thing than another takes its place. Why?

A Usually people with OCD have several obsessions or compulsions. During treatment, initially they tend gradually to get rid of the less severe obsession or compulsion and then to move on slowly to the others. Although it might sometimes seem that you are getting rid of one only for it to be replaced by another, in most cases, as time goes by, the total amount of time devoted to the rituals or obsessions will reduce.

Q I have heard that some people just get better one day. Is it true?

A OCD is in general a chronic illness. Some people may have an episodic course, which means that there is a waxing and waning of the symptoms. You should not feel guilty if the obsessions or compulsions resurface and you should continue with follow-up even if you get better since, in many cases, the dramatic changes are shortlived.

Q I have heard some people never get better, you just cope. Is it true?

A About two thirds of OCD patients get significant therapeutic response with treatment, either with medication or behaviour therapy or a combination. For the third with a more limited response a variety of other interventions might be offered (see earlier in this book for details).

Q Will pregnancy affect my OCD?

A Some studies suggest that there is an increased risk of developing OCD during pregnancy and this type of observation has led to investigation of oxytocin in the pathogenesis of OCD. However, there are some patients who claim that pregnancy is associated with a decrease or temporary disappearance of their OCD symptoms.

Q Are my children more likely to have OCD because I have it?

A Since you have experience with OCD and know the suffering that comes from the disorder not being recognized, you will be in a position to recognize OCD symptoms should they develop in your child and will be able to provide support and seek treatment early. There is some evidence of a genetic component in certain subtypes of OCD, for instance OCD with tic disorder, and possibly OCD that has very early onset. However, the mode of transmission is very different from that related to the colour of your eyes or the shape of your body and any increase in risk for the child of a parent with OCD is very slight.

Q I have noticed my child doing things that look like OCD-type behaviour. Is this OCD?

A Many very young children might have what appears to be OCD, for example not stepping on the cracks in paving stones, counting, etc. This is a natural part of growing up. Sometimes this ritualistic behaviour persists throughout puberty or begins to interfere with daily activities, or performance at school. In this case it would be worthwhile consulting an expert.

Q What should parents tell children about OCD?

A Airing problems on any subject is helpful and OCD is no different in this regard. Parents should educate their children about the disorder, emphasizing that it is a real disorder and that it does not imply the child is weak, spoiled, lacking will power, etc. If both parent and child are knowledgeable about the disorder, openly discussing the different manifestations, the research findings, the therapeutic options and the natural course, negative emotional expression about the disorder is less likely and this is associated with better prognosis.

Q What if my partner is angry because I would not do something he or she wants?

A OCD sufferers very commonly seek to involve those close to them in assisting them with carrying out rituals, or they may seek endless reassurance about their obsessions. If those close to the patient give in to these demands the OCD gets worse. It may be painful in the short term to refuse these demands but will be more helpful in the long run. The demonstration of your love and concern for your partner or your children should be expressed not by indulging the demands that are clearly related to the disorder. The doctor who is treating your partner will discuss this openly with those involved so that it is not an issue between you and your partner or child but between the patient and the physician, and you are just carrying out the doctor's orders.

Q How can I help someone with OCD when they will not get help?

A It is natural that you would like to get help for somebody who you see is suffering from his or her OCD. If the sufferer is unwilling to seek medical help it may be because he or she is afraid of the stigma of mental disorder or he or she may be sceptical about the availability of help. Many people with OCD believe they are alone in suffering their condition and tend to be very secretive about it. Learning about the disorder, its high prevalence, and the recent dramatic changes in treatment possibilities would help. Sometimes a person can be persuaded to see a specialist just for one consultation without commitment to getting into therapy, and then after appropriate explanation he or she may be ready to seek treatment.

Q Can I catch OCD symptoms if I attend a support group?

A There is no evidence that hearing of other people's symptoms can give them to you. There are even studies that suggest that the types of obsessive symptoms that run in the family are not the same. A father or mother might have washing rituals and the child checking rituals and vice versa. OCD symptoms are an integral part of the disorder, not something one learns from outside.

Q Absolutely nothing has worked. Is psychosurgery the only option?

A Before considering neurosurgery comprehensive pharmacological intervention and a thorough programme of expert behavioural therapy need to have been undertaken. There has been a great increase in the sophistication of neurosurgery, and studies of OCD patients suggest that about 30% of those who have not responded to other treatments will respond to this type of intervention.

Q Do compulsive gamblers have OCD?

A A subset of gamblers who really do not want to gamble and who derive no pleasure from gambling might have OCD. For them antiobsessive and behavioural intervention may have a place.

The relatives and friends of sufferers from OCD are often at a loss to know what they can do to help. Some families go along with the sufferer and help with the rituals; others do not actually get involved with the rituals but do not discourage them either. Sometimes they refuse to acknowledge the obsessional behaviour or they swing between being involved and refusing to have anything to do with the obsessions.

There is a great deal families can do to help:

1 Remember OCD is a treatable disorder, the symptoms are not personality traits, they are not the 'fault' of the sufferer, nor are they the fault of the family

2 Recognize the symptoms, acknowledge the OCD, and help the sufferer to recognize his or her problem as OCD

3 Encourage the sufferer to seek treatment and support his or her determination to recover

4 Learn as much as possible about the disorder and seek out information that may help the sufferer

5 Make time to allow the sufferer to explain his or her problems, as this will help the sufferer to feel less isolated

6 Encourage the sufferer to persist with treatment. Understand that there will be setbacks and do not get frustrated when they occur but do give appreciation for any improvement, however small

Cont'd.

7 Be supportive of the sufferer but do not support the obsessions and compulsions. The family can help by encouraging the sufferer to resist his or her symptoms

8 Keep the daily living routine normal and do not adapt it to accommodate the rituals or compulsion. At the same time be sensitive to the problems of the sufferer

9 Improvement in OCD may take many months. Do not expect too much too soon

10 Humour can help. OCD sufferers are often aware of the funny side of the behaviours and this can be used to help the sufferer to put distance between him or herself and the condition

Appendix:
National OCD organizations

Obsessive Action
Unit 108
Aberdeen Studios
Aberdeen Centre
22–24 Highbury Grove
London N5 2EA
UK

The OC Foundation, Inc.
PO Box 70
Milford
CT 06460
USA

OCD Association of
South Africa
PO Box 87127
Houghton 2041
Johannesburg
South Africa

Obsessive Compulsive and
Anxiety Disorders
Foundation of Victoria (Inc.)
PO Box 358
Mt Waverley
Victoria 3149
Australia

Obsessive Compulsive
Disorders Support Service
Room 318
Epworth Building
33 Pirie Street
Adelaide
SA 5000
Australia

Ananke Foundation
Mistelgatan 7
722 25 Vasteras
Sweden

International Council on OCD
Action International House
Crabtree Office Village
Eversely Way
Thorpe
Egham
UK

References

Alderman J, Wolkow R, Chung M, Johnston H. Sertraline treatment of children and adolescents with obsessive compulsive disorder or depression: Pharmacokinetics, tolerability and efficacy. *J Am Acad Child Adolesc Psychiatry* (1998) **37**: 386–94.

American Psychiatric Association. *Diagnostic and Statistical Manual of Mental Disorders (DSM-IV)* (Washington DC: APA, 1994).

Anderson IM, Tomenson BM. Treatment discontinuation with selective serotonin reuptake inhibitors compared with tricyclic antidepressants: a meta-analysis. *Br Med J* (1995) **310**: 1433–8.

Bastani B, Nash F, Meltzer HY. Prolactin and cortisol responses to MK212, a serotonin agonist, in obsessive compulsive disorder. *Arch Gen Psychiatry* (1990) **47**: 833–9.

Baxter LR, Phelps ME, Mazziotta JC, Guze BH, Schwartz JM, Selin CE. Local cerebral glucose metabolic rates in obsessive-compulsive disorder — a comparison with rates in unipolar depression and in normal controls. *Arch Gen Psychiatry* (1987) **44**: 211–18.

Baxter LR, Schwartz JM, Bergman KS et al. Caudate glucose metabolic rate changes with both drug and behaviour therapy for obsessive-compulsive disorder. *Arch Gen Psychiatry* (1992) **49**: 681–9.

Beck AT. *Cognitive Therapy and the Emotional Disorders* (New York: International University Press, 1976).

Benkelfat C, Murphy DL, Zohar J, Hill JL, Grover GN, Insel TR. Clomipramine in OCD: further evidence for a serotonergic mechanism of action. *Arch Gen Psychiatry* (1989) **46**: 23–8.

Bisserbe JC, Lane RM, Flament MF. A double-blind comparison of sertraline and clomipramine in outpatients with obsessive-compulsive disorder. *Eur Psychiatry* (1997) **12**: 82–93.

Bland RC, Newman SC, Orn HT. Period prevalence of psychiatric disorders in Edmonton. *Acta Psychiatr Scand* (1988) **77**: 24–42.

Brawman-Mintzer O, Lydiard RB, Phillips KA et al. Body dysmorphic disorder in patients with anxiety disorders and major depression: a co-morbidity study. *Am J Psychiatry* (1995) **152**: 1965–7.

Carey G, Gottesman II. Twin and family studies of anxiety, phobic and obsessive disorders. In Klein DF, Rabin J (Eds) *Anxiety: New Research and Changing Concepts* (New York: Raven Press, 1981): 117–36.

Casas M, Alvarez E, Duro P et al. Antiandrogenic treatment of obsessive-compulsive neurosis. *Acta Psychiatr Scand* (1986) **73**: 221–2.

Chen CN, Wong J, Lee N, Chan-Ho MW, Lau JT, Fung M. The Satin Community Mental Health Survey in Hong Kong II. Major findings. *Arch Gen Psychiatry* (1993) **50**: 125–33.

Chouinard G, Goodman WK, Greist JH, Jenike MA, Rasmussen SA, White K. Results of a double blind serotonin uptake inhibitor sertraline in the treatment of obsessive compulsive disorder. *Psychopharmacol Bull* (1990) **26**: 279–84.

Christensen H, Hadzi-Pavlovic D, Andrews G et al. Behaviour therapy and tricyclic medication in the treatment of obsessive-compulsive disorder: a quantitative review. *J Consult Clin Psychol* (1987) **55**: 701–11.

Cohen DJ, Dexter J, Young G et al. Clonidine ameliorates Gilles de la Tourette syndrome. *Arch Gen Psychiatry* (1980) **37**: 1350–7.

Cottraux J, Mollard E, Bouvard M et al. A controlled study of fluvoxamine and exposure in obsessive compulsive disorders. *Int Clin Psychopharmacol* (1990) **5**: 17–30.

Cox BJ, Swinson RP. Clomipramine, fluoxetine, and behavior therapy in the treatment of obsessive-compulsive disorder: a meta-analysis. *J Behav Ther Experi Psychiat* (1993) **24**: 149–53.

Degonda M, Wyss M, Angst J. The Zurich Study. XVIII. Obsessive compulsive disorders and syndromes in the general population. *Eur Arch Psychiat Clin Neurosci* (1993) **243**: 16–22.

de Veaugh Geiss J, Landau P, Katz RJ. Treatment of obsessive compulsive disorder with clomipramine. *Psychiatr Ann* (1989) **19**: 97–101.

de Veaugh Geiss J, Moroz G, Biederman J et al. Clomipramine hydrochloride in childhood and adolescent obsessive-compulsive disorder: a multicentre trial. *J Am Acad Child Adolesc Psychiatr* (1992) **31**: 45–9.

Dunbar GC, Steiner M, Bushnell WD. Long-term treatment and prevention of relapse of obsessive compulsive disorder with paroxetine. *Eur Neuropsychopharmacol* (1995) **5**: 372 (abstract).

Emmelkamp PMG, Kwee K. Obsessional ruinations: a comparison between thought-stopping and prolonged exposure in imagination. *Behav Res Ther* (1977) **15**: 441–4.

Emmelkamp PMG, Visser S, Hoekstra RJ. Cognitive therapy vs exposure in vivo in the treatment of obsessive-compulsives. *Cogn Ther Res* (1988) **12**: 103–14.

Fallon BA, Campeas R, Schneier FR et al. Open trial of intravenous clomipramine in five treatment refractory patients with obsessive compulsive disorder. *J Neuropsychiatry* (1992) **4**: 70–5.

Fallon BA, Liebowitz MR, Salmon E et al. Fluoxetine for hypochondriacal patients without major depression. *J Clin Psychopharmacol* (1993) **13**: 438–41.

Fernandez CE, Lopez-Ibor JJ. Monochlorimipramine in the treatment of psychiatric patients resistant to other therapies. *Actas Luso Esp Neuro Psiquiatr Cienc* (1967) **26**: 119–47.

Fineberg NA. Refining treatment approaches in obsessive-compulsive disorder. *Int Clin Psychopharmacol* (1996) **11**: 13–22.

Flament MF, Rapoport JL, Berg CJ. Clomipramine treatment of childhood OCD: a double-blind controlled study. *Arch Gen Psychiatry* (1985) **42**: 977–83.

Flament MF, Rapoport JL, Murphy DL, Berg CJ, Lake CR. Biochemical changes during clomipramine treatment of childhood OCD. *Arch Gen Psychiatry* (1987) **44**: 219–25.

Flament MF, Whitaker A, Rapoport JL et al. Obsessive compulsive disorder in adolescence: an epidemiological study *J Am Acad Child Adolesc Psychiatr* (1988) **27**: 764–71.

Foa E, Steketee G, Ozarow BJ. Behaviour therapy with obsessive-compulsives: from theory to treatment. In Mavissakalian M, Turner SM, Michelson L (Eds) *Obsessive-Compulsive Disorder: Psychological and Pharmacological Treatment* (New York: Plenum Press, 1985): 49–129.

Frankel M, Cummings JL, Robertson MM, Trimble MR, Hill MA, Benson DF. Obsessions and compulsions in Gilles de la Tourette's syndrome. *Neurology* (1986) **36**: 378–82.

Freeman CP, Trimble MR, Deakin JFW et al. Fluvoxamine or clomipramine in the treatment of obsessive-compulsive disorder? A multicenter, randomized double-blind, parallel group comparison. *J Clin Psychiat* (1994) **55**: 301–5.

Goodman WK, Kozak MJ, Liebowitz M, White KL. Treatment of obsessive-compulsive disorder with fluvoxamine: a multicentre, double-blind, placebo-controlled trial. *Int Clin Psychopharmacol* (1996) **11**: 21–30.

Goodman WK, McDougle CJ, Barr LC et al. Biological approaches to treatment-resistant obsessive compulsive disorder. *J Clin Psych* (1993) **54**: 16–26.

Goodman WK, Price LH, Delgado PL et al. Specificity of serotonin reuptake inhibitors in the treatment of obsessive compulsive disorder: comparison of fluvoxamine and desipramine. *Arch Gen Psychiatry* (1990) **47**: 577–85.

Goodman WK, Price LH, Rasmussen SA, Delgado PL, Heninger GR, Charney DS. Efficacy of fluvoxamine in obsessive compulsive disorder. *Arch Gen Psychiatry* (1989) **46**: 36–44.

Greist JH, Chouinard G, DuBoff E et al. Double-blind parallel comparison of three dosages of sertraline and placebo in outpatients with obsessive-compulsive disorder. *Arch Gen Psychiatry* (1995c) **52**: 289–95.

Greist JH, Jefferson JW, Kobak KA et al. A 1 year double-blind placebo-controlled fixed dose study of sertraline in the treatment of obsessive-compulsive disorder. *Int Clin Psychopharmacol* (1995a) **10**: 57–65.

Greist JH, Jefferson JW, Kobak KA, Katzelnick DJ, Serlin RC. Efficacy and tolerability of serotonin transport inhibitors in obsessive-compulsive disorder. *Arch Gen Psychiatry* (1995b) **52**: 53–60.

Griest JH, Jenike MA, Robinson DS, Rasmussen SA. Efficacy of fluvoxamine in obsessive-compulsive disorder: results of a multicentre, double blind, placebo-controlled trial. *Eur J Clin Res* (1995d) **7**: 195–204.

Hewlett WA, Vinogradov S, Agras WS. Clomipramine, clonazepam, and clonidine treatment of obsessive compulsive disorder. *J Clin Psychopharmacol* (1992) **12**: 420–30.

Hiss H, Foa E, Kozak MJ. Relapse prevention programme for treatment of obsessive-compulsive disorder. *J Consult Clin Psychol* (1994) **62**: 801–8.

Hodgson R, Marks IM. The treatment of obsessive compulsive neurosis: follow up and further findings. *Behav Res Ther* (1972) **10**: 181–9.

Hoehn-Saric R, Harrison W, Clary C. Obsessive compulsive disorder with comorbid major depression: a comparison of sertraline and desipramine treatment. *Eur Psychopharmacol* (1997) **7**: S180.

Hollander E. Obsessive-compulsive disorder-related disorders: the role of selective serotonergic reuptake inhibitors. *Int Clin Psychopharmacol* (1996) **11**: 75–87.

Hollander E, DeCaria CM, Nitesai A et al. Serotonergic function in obsessive compulsive disorder: behavioural and neuroendocrine responses to oral m-chlorophenylpiperazine and fenfluramine in patients and normal volunteers. *Arch Gen Psychiatry* (1992) **42**: 21–8.

Hollander E, Fay M, Liebowitz MR et al. Clonidine and clomipramine in obsessive-compulsive-disorder. *Am J Psychiatry* (1988) **145**: 388–9.

Hollander E, Greenwald S, Neville D et al. Uncomplicated and comorbid obsessive-compulsive disorder in an epidemiologic sample. *Depression and Anxiety* (1997) **4**: 111–19.

Hollander E, Liebowitz M. Augmentation of antiobsessional treatment with fenfluramine. *Am J Psychiatry* (1988) **145**: 1314–15.

Hollander E, Liebowitz MR, DeCaria CM et al. Treatment of depersonalization with serotonin re-uptake blockers. *J Clin Psychopharmacol* (1990) **10**: 200–3.

Hollander E, Wong CM. Introduction: obsessive-compulsive spectrum disorders. *J Clin Psychiatry* (1995) **56**: 3–6.

Insel TR, Akiskal HS. Obsessive compulsive disorder with psychotic features: a phenomenologic analysis. *Am J Psychiatry* (1986) **143**: 1527–33.

Insel TR, Murphy DL, Cohen RM, Alterman I, Kilts C, Linnoila M. Obsessive compulsive disorder — a double blind trial of clomipramine and clorgyline. *Arch Gen Psychiatry* (1983) **40**: 605–12.

Janet P. *Les obsessions et la psychasthénie, Volume 1* (Paris: Alcon, 1903). Cited in Pitman RK. Pierre Janet on obsessive compulsive disorder, 1903. Review and commmentary. *Arch Gen Psych* (1987) **44**: 226–32.

Jaskari MO. Observations on mianserin in the treatment of obsessive neuroses. *Curr Med Res Opin* (1980) **6**: 128–31.

Jenike MA, Baer L, Minichiello WE, Rauch SL, Buttolph ML. Placebo-controlled trial of fluoxetine and phenelzine for obsessive-compulsive disorder. *Am J Psychiatry* (1997) **154**: 1261–4.

Judd FK, Chua P, Lynch C et al. Fenfluramine augmentation of clomipramine treatment of obsessive compulsive disorder. *Aust J Psychiatry* (1991) **25**: 412–14.

Karno M, Golding JM. Obsessive compulsive disorder. In Robins LN, Regier DA (Eds) *Psychiatric Disorders in America. The Epidemiologic Catchment Area Study* (London: Macmillan, 1991): 204–19.

Karno M, Golding J, Sorenson S, Burnam MA. The epidemiology of obsessive compulsive disorder in five US communities. *Arch Gen Psychiatry* (1988) **49**: 1094–9.

Katz RJ, de Veaugh Geiss J, Landau P. Clomipramine in obsessive compulsive disorder. *Biol Psychiatry* (1990) **28**: 401–4.

Kaye WH, Weltzin TE, Hsu L. Anorexia nervosa. In Hollander E (Ed) *Obsessive-Compulsive Related Disorders* (Washington, DC: American Psychiatry Press, 1993): 49–70.

Anonymous. Epidemiology of obsessive compulsive disorder in India.

Kirk J. Behavioural treatment of obsessional-compulsive patients in routine clinical practice. *Behav Res Ther* (1983) **21**: 57–62.

Knesevich JW. Successful treatment of obsessive compulsive disorder with clonidine hydrochloride. *Am J Psychiatry* (1982) **139**: 364–5.

Koran LM, McElroy SL, Davidson JRT, Rasmussen SA, Hollander E, Jenike MA. Fluvoxamine versus clomipramine for obsessive-compulsive disorder: a double-blind comparison. *J Clin Psychiatry* (1996) **16**: 121–9.

Kronig M, Apter J, Asnis G et al. A multicentre trial of sertraline for obsessive-compulsive disorder. *Am Col Neuropsychopharmacol* (1994) (abstract).

Leonard HL, Swedo SE, Rapoport JL, Coffey M, Cheslow DL. Treatment of childhood obsessive compulsive disorder with clomipramine and desmethylimipramine: a double blind crossover comparison. *Psychopharmacol Bull* (1988) **24**: 93–5.

Leonard HL, Swedo SE, Lenane MC, et al. A double-blind desipramine substitution during long-term clomipramine treatment in children and adolescents with obsessive compulsive disorder. *Arch Gen Psychiatry* (1991) **48**: 922–7.

Lesch KP, Hoh A, Disselkamp-Tietze J, Weissman MM, Osterheider M, Schult E. 5-hydroxytryptamine 1A receptor responsivity in obsessive compulsive disorder. Comparison of patients and controls. *Arch Gen Psychiatry* (1991) **48 (suppl 6)**: 540–7.

Lindal E, Stefansson JG. The lifetime prevalence of anxiety disorders in Iceland as estimated by the US National Institute of Mental Health Diagnostic Interview Schedule. *Acta Psychiatr Scand* (1993) 29–34.

Lindsay M, Crino R, Andrews G. Controlled trial of exposure and response prevention in obsessive-compulsive disorder. *Br J Psychiatry* (1997) **171**: 135–9.

Lopez-Ibor JJ, Saiz J, Cottraux J et al. Double-blind comparison of fluoxetine versus clomipramine in the treatment of obsessive compulsive disorder. *Eur Neuropsychopharmacol* (1996) **6**: 111–18.

Luxenberg JS, Swedo SE, Flament MF, Friedland RP, Rapoport JL, Rapoport SI. Neuroanatomical abnormalities in obsessive-compulsive disorder determined with quantitative x-ray computed tomography. *Am J Psychiatry* (1988) **145**: 1089–95.

Maletsky B, McFarland B, Bart A. Refractory obsessive-compulsive disorder and ECT. *Convulsive Ther* (1994) **10**: 34–42.

Marazziti D, Hollander E, Lensi P et al. Peripheral markers of serotonin and dopamine function in obsessive-compulsive disorder. *Psychiatr Res* (1992) **42**: 41–51.

March JS, Biederman J, Wolkow R et al. Sertraline in children and adults with obsessive-compulsive disorder: a multicenter randomized controlled trial. *JAMA* (1998) **280**: 1752–6.

Markovitz PJ, Stagno SJ, Calabrese JR. Buspirone augmentation of fluoxetine on obsessive-compulsive disorder. *Am J Psychiatry* (1990) **147**: 798–800.

Marks IM, Hodgson R, Rachman S. Treatment of chronic obsessive compulsive neurosis by in vivo exposure. *Br J Psychiatry* (1975) 127: 349–64.

Marks IM, Lelliott P, Basoglu M et al. Clomipramine, self exposure and therapist aided exposure for obsessive compulsive rituals. *Br J Psychiatry* (1988) **152**: 522–34.

Marks IM, Stern RS, Mawson D, Cobb J, McDonald R. Clomipramine and exposure for obsessive compulsive rituals. *Br J Psychiatry* (1980) **136**: 1–25.

Mavissakalian M, Turner S, Michelson L, Jacob R. Tricyclic antidepressants in obsessive disorder: antiobsessional or antidepressant agents. *Am J Psychiatry* (1985) **142**: 572–6.

McDougle CJ, Barr LC, Goodman WK et al. Lack of efficacy of clozapine monotherapy in refractory obsessive-compulsive disorder. *Am J Psychiatry* (1995a) **152**: 1812–14.

McDougle CJ, Fleischmann RL, Epperson CN, Wasyling S, Leckman JF, Price LH. Risperidone addition in fluvoxamine-refractory obsessive-compulsive disorder: three cases. *J Clin Psychiatry* (1995b) **56**: 526–8.

McDougle CJ, Goodman WK, Leckman JF et al. Limited therapeutic effect of addition of buspirone in fluvoxamine-refractory obsessive compulsive disorder. *Am J Psychiatry* (1993) **150**: 647–9.

McDougle CJ, Goodman WK, Price LH et al. Neuroleptic addition in fluvoxamine-refractory obsessive-compulsive disorder. *Am J Psychiatry* (1990) **147**: 652–4.

McDougle CJ, Price LH, Goodman WK, Charney DS, Heninger GR. A controlled trial of lithium augmentation in fluvoxamine refractory obsessive-compulsive disorders lack of efficacy. *J Clin Psychopharmacol* (1991) **11**: 175–84.

McElroy SL, Phillips KA, Keck PE. Obsessive-compulsive spectrum disorder. *J Clin Psychiatry* (1994) **55**: 33–51.

McKay D, Todaro J, Neziroglu F, Yaryura-Tobias JA. Evaluation of a naturalistic maintenance program in the treatment of obsessive-compulsive disorder: a preliminary investigation. *J Anx Dis* (1996) **10**: 211–17.

Meyer V. Modification of expectations in cases with obsessional rituals. *Behav Res Ther* (1996) **4**: 273–80.

Milanfranchi A, Ravagli S, Lensi P, Marazziti D, Cassano GB. A double-blind study of fluvoxamine and clomipramine in the treatment of obsessive-compulsive disorder. *Int Clin Psychopharmacol* (1997) **12**: 131–6.

Montgomery SA. Clomipramine in obsessional neurosis: a placebo controlled trial. *Pharmaceut Med* (1980) **1**: 189–92.

Montgomery SA, Fineberg NA, Montgomery DB, Bullock T. L-tryptophan in obsessive compulsive disorder — a placebo controlled study. *Eur Neuropsychopharmacol* (1992) **2 (suppl 2)**: 384.

Montgomery SA, Henry J, McDonald G et al. Selective serotonin reuptake inhibitors: meta-analysis of discontinuation rate. *Int Clin Psychopharmacol* (1994) **9**: 47–53.

Montgomery SA, Kasper S. Comparison of compliance between serotinin reuptake inhibitors and tricyclic antidepressants: a meta-analysis. *Int Clin Psychopharmacol* (1995) **9 (suppl 4)**: 33–40.

Montgomery SA, McIntyre A, Osterheider M et al. and the Lilly European OCD Study Group. A double-blind, placebo-controlled study of fluoxetine in patients with DSM-III-R obsessive compulsive disorder. *Eur Neuropsychopharmacol* (1993) **3**: 143–52.

Montgomery SA. Citalopram treatment of obsessive compulsive disorder: results from a double-blind placebo-controlled study. Presented at the 37th Annual Meeting of the American College of Neuropsychopharmacology, Las Croaloas, Puerto Rico, December 1998.

Okasha A, Saad A, Khalil AM et al. Phenomenology of OCD. A transcultural study. *Comp Psychiat* (1994) **35**: 191–7.

Pato M, Hill JL, Murphy DL. A clomlipramine dosage reduction study in the course of long-term treatment of obsessive-compulsive disorder patients. *Psychopharmacol Bull* (1990) **26**: 211–14.

Pato M, Pigott TA, Hill JL, Grover GN, Bernstein SE, Murphy DL. Controlled comparison of buspirone and clomipramine in obsessive-compulsive disorder. *Am J Psychiatry* (1991) **148**: 127–9.

Pato M, Zohar-Kadouch R, Zohar J, Murphy DL. Return of symptoms after discontinuation of clomipramine in patients with obsessive compulsive disorder. *Am J Psychiatry* (1988) **145**: 1543–8.

Pauls DL, Alsobrook J, Goodman WK et al. A family study of obsessive-compulsive disorder. *Am J Psychiatry* (1995) **152**: 76–84.

Pauls DL, Towbin KE, Leckerman JF et al. Gilles de la Tourette's syndrome and obsessive-compulsive disorder: evidence supporting a genetic relationship. *Arch Gen Psychiatry* (1986) **43**: 1180–2.

Perse TL, Greist JH, Jefferson JW, Rosenfeld JW, Dar R. Fluvoxamine treatment of obsessive compulsive disorder. *Am J Psychiatry* (1987) **144**: 1543–8.

Piccinelli M, Pini S, Bellantuono C, Wilkinson G. Efficacy of drug treatment in obsessive-compulsive disorder. *Br J Psychiatry* (1995) **166**: 424–43.

Pigott TA, Pato M, Bernstein SE et al. Controlled comparison of clomipramine and fluoxetine in the treatment of obsessive-compulsive disorder. *Arch Gen Psychiatry* (1990) **47**: 926–32.

Pigott TA, Pato M, L'Heureux F. A controlled comparison of adjuvant lithium carbonate or thyroid hormone in clomipramine-treated OCD patients. *J Clin Psychopharmacol* (1991) **11**: 245–8.

Pigott TA, L'Heureux F, Rubenstein CS, Bernstein SE, Hill JL, Murphy DL. A double-blind placebo controlled study of trazodone in patients with obsessive-compulsive disorder. *J Clin Psychopharmacol* (1992) **12**: 156–62.

Pitman RK, Green RC, Jenike MA, Mesulam MM. Clinical comparison of Tourette's disorder and obsessive-compulsive disorder. *Am J Psychiatry* (1987) **144**: 1166–71.

Rachman S. The modification of obsessions: a new formulation. *Behav Res Ther* (1976) **14**: 443.

Rachman S, Hodgson R. *Obsessions and Compulsions* (New York: Prentice-Hall, 1980).

Rachman S, Hodgson R, Marks IM. Treatment of chronic obsessive compulsive neuroses. *Behav Res Ther* (1971) **9**: 237–47.

Rachman S, Marks IM, Hodgson R. The treatment of obsessive compulsive neurotics by modelling and flooding in vivo. *Behav Res Ther* (1973) **11**: 463–71.

Rasmussen SA, Eisen JL. Clinical and epidemiologic findings of significance to neuropharmacologic trials in OCD. *Psychopharmacol Bull* (1988) **24**: 466–70.

Rasmussen S, Eisen J. The epidemiology and clinical features of obsessive-compulsive disorder. *Psychiatr Clin North Am* (1992) **14**: 743–58.

Rasmussen S, Hacket E, DuBoff E et al. A 2-year study of sertraline in the treatment of obsessive-compulsive disorder *Int Clin Psychopharmacol* (1997) **12**: 309–16.

Rasmussen SA, Tsuang MT. The epidemiology of obsessive compulsive disorder. *J Clin Psychiatry* (1984) **45**: 450–7.

Rasmussen SA, Tsuang MT. Clinical characteristics and family history in DSM-III obsessive compulsive disorder *Am J Psychiatry* (1986) **143**: 317–22.

Rauch SL, Jenike MA. Management of treatment-resistant obsessive compulsive disorder: concepts and strategies. In Hollander E, Zohar J, Marazziti D (eds) *Current Insights in Obsessive Compulsive Disorder* (Chichester: Wiley, 1994): 227–44.

Rauch SL, Jenike MA, Alpert NM et al. Regional cerebral blood flow measured during symptom provocation in obsessive-compulsive disorder using 150-labeled CO_2 and positron emission tomography. *Arch Gen Psychiatry* (1994) **51**: 62–70.

Rauch SL, O'Sullivan RL, Jenike MA. Open treatment of obsessive-compulsive disorder with venlafaxine: a series of ten cases. *J Clin Psychopharmacol* (1998) **16**: 81–3.

Reinherz HZ, Giaconia RM, Lefkowitz ES, Pakiz B, Frost AK. Prevalence of psychiatric disorders in a community population of older adolescents. *J Am Acad Child Adolesc Psychiatr* (1993) **32**: 69–77.

Remington G, Adams M. Risperidone and obsessive-compulsive symptoms. *J Clin Psychopharmacol* (1994) **14**: 358–9 (letter).

Riddle MA, Scahill L, King RA et al. Double-blind, crossover trial of fluoxetine and placebo in children and adolescents with obsessive-compulsive disorder. *J Am Acad Child Adolesc Psychiatr* (1992) **31**: 1062–9.

Roberts JM, Lydiard RB. Sertraline for bulimia nervosa (case history). *Am J Psychiatry* (1994) **150**: 1753.

Robins LN, Helzer JE, Weissman M et al. Lifetime prevalence of specific psychiatric disorders in three sites. *Arch Gen Psychiatry* (1984) **138**: 949–58.

Roper G, Rachman S, Marks IM. Passive and participant modelling in exposure treatment of obsessive compulsive neurotics. *Behav Res Ther* (1975) **13**: 271–9.

Rothenburg A. Adolescence and eating disorders: the obsessive-compulsive syndrome. *Psychiat Clin N Am* (1990) **13**: 469–88.

Rubenstein CS, Pigott TA, L'Heureux F et al. A preliminary investigation of the lifetime prevalence of anorexia and bulimia nervosa in patients with obsessive-compulsive disorder. *J Clin Psychiatry* (1992) **53**: 309–14.

Salkovskis PM. Obsessional-compulsive problems: a cognitive-behavioural analysis. *Behav Res Ther* (1985) **23**: 571–83.

Scarone S, Colombo C, Livian S et al. Increased right caudate nucleus size in obsessive compulsive disorder. *Psychia Res Neuroimaging* (1992) **45**: 115–21.

Smeraldi E, Erzegovesi S, Bianchi I et al. Fluvoxamine v. clomipramine treatment in obsessive-compulsive disorder: a preliminary study. *New Trends Exp Clin Psych* (1992) **8**: 63–5.

Stein DJ, Hollander E. Low-dose pimozide augmentation of serotonin re-uptake blockers in the treatment of trichotillomania. *J Clin Psychiatry* (1993) **53**: 123–6.

Swedo SE, Leonard HL, Rapoport JL et al. A double-blind comparison of clomipramine and desipramine in the treatment of trichotillomania (hair-pulling). *N Eng J Med* (1989) **321**: 497–501.

Swedo SE, Leonard HL, Shapiro MB et al. Sydenham's chorea: physical and psychological symptoms of St Vitus' dance. *Paediatrics* (1993) **91**: 706–13.

Thoren P, Asberg M, Bertilsson L, Mellstrom B, Sjoqvist F, Traskman L. Clomipramine treatment of obsessive compulsive disorder. II. Biochemical aspects. *Arch Gen Psychiatry* (1980a) **37**: 1289–94.

Thoren P, Asberg M, Cronholm B, Jornestedt L, Traskman L. Clomipramine treatment in obsessive compulsive disorder. I. A controlled clinical trial. *Arch Gen Psychiatry* (1980b) **37**: 1281–5.

Tollefson GD, Rampey AH, Potvin JH et al. A multicenter investigation of fixed-dose fluoxetine in the treatment of obsessive-compulsive disorder. *Arch Gen Psychiatry* (1994) **51**: 559–67.

Vallejo J, Olivares J, Marcos TI Bulbena A, Menchon JM. Clomipramine versus phenelzine in obsessive compulsive disorder. A controlled clinical trial. *Br J Psychiatry* (1992) **161**: 665–70.

Valleni-Basile LA, Garrison CZ, Jackson KL et al. Frequency of obsessive compulsive disorder in a community sample of young adolescents. *J Am Acad Child Adolesc Psychiatr* (1994) **33**: 782–91.

van Balkom AJLM, van Oppen, Vermulen AWA et al. A meta-analysis on the treatment of obsessive-compulsive disorder: a comparison of antidepressants, behaviour, and cognitive therapy. *Clin Psychol Rev* (1994) **14**: 359–81.

van Oppen P, de Haan E, van Balkom AJLM et al. Cognitive therapy and exposure in vivo in the treatment of obsessive-compulsive disorder. *Behav Res Ther* (1995) **33**: 379–90.

Warneke L. Intravenous chlorimipramine therapy in obsessive compulsive disorder. *Can J Psychiatry* (1989) 34: 853–9.

Weissman MM, Bland RC, Canino GL et al. The Cross National Epidemiology of Obsessive-Compulsive Disorder. *J Clin Psychiat* (1994) **55**: 5–10.

Wheadon D, Bushnell WD, Steiner M. A fixed dose comparison of 20, 40 or 60 mg of paroxetine to placebo in the treatment of obsessive-compulsive disorder. *ACNP* (abstract).

Wood A. Pharmacotherapy of bulimia nervosa — experience with fluoxetine. *Int Clin Psychopharmacol* (1993) **8**: 259–301.

Wood A, Tollefson GD, Birkett M. Pharmacotherapy of obsessive compulsive disorder experience with fluoxetine. *Int Clin Psychopharmacol* (1993) **8**: 301–6.

Zohar AH, Ratzoni G, Pauls DL et al. An epidemiological study of obsessive compulsive disorder and related disorders in Israeli adolescents. *J Am Acad Child Adolesc Psychiatr* (1992a) **31**: 1057–61.

Zohar J. Is 5-HT1D involved in obsessive-compulsive disorder? *Eur Neuropsychopharmacol* (1996) **6**: 55.

Zohar J, Insel TR. Obsessive compulsive disorder: psychobiological approaches to diagnosis, treatment and pathophysiology. *Biol Psychiatry* (1987) **22**: 667–87.

Zohar J, Judge R. Paroxetine versus clomipramine in the treatment of obsessive-compulsive disorder. *Br J Psychiatry* (1996) **169**: 468–74.

Zohar J, Zohar-Kadouch R, Kindler S. Current concepts in the pharmacological treatment of obsessive compulsive disorder. *Drugs* (1992b) **43**: 218.

Index

Note: page numbers in *italics* refer to figures and tables